THE BODYTALK

JUDY COLE

HEAL YOUR WEIGHT

STOP DIGGING YOUR GRAVE WITH YOUR KNIFE & FORK

Dedicated to my parents, with love

"The doctor of the future will give no medicine, but will interest his patients in the care of the human body, in diet and in the cause and prevention of disease."

Thomas Alva Edison
1847-1931

THE BODYTALKS

JUDY COLE

HEAL YOUR WEIGHT

STOP DIGGING YOUR GRAVE WITH YOUR KNIFE & FORK

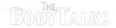

Published by Alchemist Publishing International.

Alchemist Publishing, UK
1-18 Hams Crescent
Knightbridge
London
SW1X OLL

www.judycole.co.uk
judy@judycole.co.uk
www.thebodytalks.com

First published 2003
First re-print 2004

Copyright: Judy Cole
Design Copyright: Judy Cole

ISBN 0-9546950-0-3

All rights reserved. No part of this publication may be reproduced in any material form (including photography or storing in any medium by electronic means) without the written permission of the copyright holder. Applications for the copyright holders written permission to reproduce any part of this publication should be addressed to the publishe Any person acting in contravention of this copyright will be liable to criminal prosecution and the civil claims for damages.

Designed by Jonathan Court and Judy Cole
Photographs by Nick Crawley

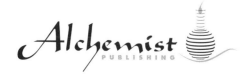

CONTENTS

	About the Author	6
	How to use this book	10
1	Stop all this diet nonsense	14
2	Food Intolerances	22
3	Food Basics: Proteins, Carbs, Fats, Cholesterol & Insulin	44
4	Rules of good eating	72
	The Programme:	92
5	Stage 1. The Detox	93
6	Stage 2. The Healing	108
7	Stage 3. The Maintenance	114
8	Eating Out	118
9	Supplements	128
10	A-Z of useful Information	134
11	Liver Cleanse	150
12	The Complications: Thyroid & Candida	155
13	Recipes	166
	Recommended reading	186
	Acknowledgements	187
	Index	188

About the Author

I am more surprised than anyone to be writing this book. Looking back now, it has been a journey that began many years ago, and I think I always had its purpose in this end. Or is it the beginning? This book is the culmination of the past twenty four years, starting with the first awareness of being slightly overweight at the age of ten, and the first attempt to watch what I ate. I was a chubby child, particularly in my legs and hips, which became, as I grew into my teens, the bane of my life. I now know, at the wise old age of thirty five, that that unwanted weight was not a result of overeating: my mother fed me very well. It was the beginning signs of toxic build up of foods which my particular genetic body was unable to process. Every time I ate these common everyday foods, my immune system thought it was under attack from an enemy invader, a little like a bacteria or virus. Launched repeatedly to fight the invader, the adrenal glands and immune system slowly became more and more exhausted from the continual onslaught. In the meantime, tiny residues that the body could not eliminate, began to accumulate in 'safe' areas of my body away from vital organs, particularly the hips and thighs. I had cellulite at twelve years old!! Just how unfair could that be? Nor was it a toxic environment. I was fortunate enough to be born and brought up in the relatively unpolluted and non industrialised country of Zambia, in Africa, where most of the foods were grown locally and without excessive insecticides or processing and brought fresh to market. The shortages of imported foodstuffs meant we had little access to junk and processed foods, a terrible deprivation for a child aware of what was available during intermittent trips to the UK and abroad, but a blessing in disguise in retrospect. Looking back now I was a sluggish child, I yawned a lot and remember people often asking me why I was bored. I was unaware I was even doing it but now notice how within a few minutes of eating one of my food intolerances, I begin to yawn. I could never wake up in the mornings, feeling like I had a fog in my brain for the first few hours every morning and school was a huge effort. When you don't know any better, you assume you are normal, maybe just a tad lazy or something, but just a normal kid. Only now, basking in the glorious new found superhealth of a food intolerance free life, do I realise what a handicap the effects of those foods gave me growing up. It all came to a head when I was twenty five years old.

At the time I was working as a sports injury and remedial massage specialist with professional sports teams, athletes and ballet dancers in the UK. I had just completed a masters degree in sport science at Leeds Metropolitan University.

During the preceeding six years I had been working in top professional sport as one of Britain's first full time remedial massage specialists with clients that included the England Cricket Team, Leeds United AFC, Torvill and Dean, the Olympic ice skaters and the Northern Ballet Theatre. During those years I met and studied with a brilliant Chinese master masseur whose patience and skill taught me to read the body with my hands and manipulate energy blocks. He showed me how to feel new and old injury, trauma areas which resulted in stagnant chi and to follow the line of injury to its true source. I am eternally grateful to Mr Kai Chi.

Then in January 1995, I suffered a bad attack of numbness down the left side of my body, over the next two months I slowly lost the use, control and feeling in my left leg. In March I was diagnosed with Multiple Sclerosis.

In a quest to cure the illness, my search led me to nutrition and kinesiology. I discovered that the whole basis of my illness was due to food intolerances or foods which my genetically sensitive B blood type body could not digest and recognise as nutritional. Instead, these foods had had an insidious and devastating affect on my brain and brain chemistry over time. In 1995, very few people understood the impact of food intolerances, but as a result of my experience and eventual resulting cure of this devastating disease, I began to research further into the unknown area of the more subtle impact of food on our bodies.

In 1995, needing to escape the British weather, still numb in one side and weak in my left leg, I decided to move to Dubai, a good compromise between the warmth and freedom of my youth in Africa, and the more sophisticated lifestyle I had grown accustomed to in the UK. During the following two years, I set up a part time practice, working with kinesiology and sports injuries. I began to explore the relationship that injuries had to food. In 1998, I felt a deep need to return to my African roots, and moved down to South Africa to live in the beautiful area of Plettenberg Bay, on the south coast.

I spent a wonderful eighteen months down there, nurturing my spiritual growth and meeting some very special teachers, who awakened in me a gift for dowsing. Dowsing is an ability to use a pendulum to talk to the universal all knowingness, which includes the ability to dowse for water and oil and to 'talk' to the body through tuning into the energy of a person and asking their bodies about their health. It has taken me four years to trust this system, only after seeing results prove its accuracy. In the meantime I found I was also able to use the skill of muscle testing, a method learned during the study of kinesiology, to ask the body things about itself with an extraordinary accuracy. I returned to Dubai and set up a full time practice.

I began to ask the body more direct questions, particularly about nutrition and health and, encouraged by the outcome, found I could ask the body anything I wanted about its physical, mental and emotional health. With my insatiable underlying curiosity to find out why and how we got ill, my experience grew and the successive positive results with my clients has built up an incredibly busy practice with people seeking help from all over the world, about illnesses and conditions that conventional medicine could not help. In the last four years I have treated over 2000 people and have a conservative estimate of more than 1500 cases where clients have either cured or improved dramatically from problems that conventional medicine had failed either to diagnose or help. I have found there is no limit to what a body could tell me about illness, nutrition, disease and how the body could heal itself. The questions were limited by my understanding of the body, biology and healing. Often the body explained illnesses and conditions as being very different from established medical theory and further proved itself by healing when that body's theory was adopted and used to treat the condition.

It became increasingly evident that the most important basis for healing was the elimination of food from the diet to which your body was intolerant to and the adoption of correct balanced nutrition, before the overburdened immune system could be strengthened enough to heal any other condition. In fact, I would estimate that nearly fifty percent of the problems I see are directly caused by food intolerances themselves. Many of the case histories in this book will illustrate this.

This book is therefore the direct result of the body's teachings on how and what we need to eat to be healthy. The information has come directly from asking the body, through personal experience and successful results, with those wonderful, trusting, dedicated clients.

Five years ago, many of the premises of The Body Talks Programme were revolutionary and went against many of the accepted nutritional rules of the past two decades. But the results spoke for themselves, as did the basic common sense of the information the body revealed.

Quite simply, it works.

It works because our bodies know what they need, as individuals and as a biological human being. It recognises that we have evolved with our environment and our cultures through generations, to adapt to new foods and ways of eating. It illustrates how our blood type influences the way we react to different food, explaining why you can eat one thing that makes another person ill. The programme is a return, to nature, to good sense, to balanced simple eating. It is firmly based in the realities of busy modern life.

When we meet and connect either in person or through this book, I share the onus of helping you find your health. But I do not do it alone. I need three specific inputs from you.

Faith and an open mind to listen to what I am saying
Will power to put it into action
And
Self love, patience and commitment to make it a reality.

Oh, and when you make it, please spare me a thought - drop me an e-mail and we can toast your new self together. I wish you bon voyage, finding your health and ideal body, for life is a wonderful journey.
Enjoy your journey of self discovery!

Judy Cole.
Dubai 2003

www.judycole.co.uk					www.thebodytalks.com

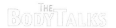

HOW TO USE THIS BOOK

This book is a manual for healing your weight by good eating habits over three to six months, and in the process, reclaiming your life-given right to superhealth and vitality. It is not a quick fix diet and should NOT be undertaken as such. It requires a commitment to yourself and recognises that years of abuse must be reversed slowly and cannot be changed overnight.

Nor have I blinded you with science. I have tried to enlighten you as to how nutrition really works and give you simplified but realistic models that explain the underlying basic processes of digestion. These can then be applied easily to your everyday eating habits. The Body Talks rules are basic common sense outlined to me by the body but which are also evident through more recent scientific research into nutrition and biology. Each element of this programme can be further investigated in recent books that explain each of them in greater scientific detail and have been published only in the last few years. But each book has only addressed one issue and it is all of these that must be brought together to complete the puzzle of truly healthy eating for life. These are listed at the back of the book for further reading. From these books I was able to understand more deeply what the body was trying to tell me and this programme recognises their contribution.

The first chapters give you all the information you really need about food so you can learn to make informed balanced choices about what you eat for the rest of your life. In Chapter 5, 6 and 7 there are easy to follow dietplans for each stage of your recovery, which give you complete choice to follow your own likes and dislikes within cultural limitations.

Read the book right through before you begin and mark areas that emphasise points that will be needed by you again and again during your programme. Make sure you understand all the principles. Prepare your kitchen and tell people you are embarking on a new way of life. Enlist their support and encouragement. Your progress may inspire many others to follow your example.

"What? You mean I'm not meant to be fat?" was my startled reaction to Judy's diagnosis. "No, you're just not eating right for your type" said Judy. You see, I'd always been fat; I'd been fat all my life and over the last couple of years I'd got really fat-92kg fat. About eight months before I met Judy I'd attacked the problem like never before, doing regular supervised work-outs in the gym and eating 'healthily'. I'd lost a lot of weight, but couldn't seem to lose any more. This was when I met Judy. She told me that the kinds of 'healthy' foods I was eating-lots of pasta with tomato sauce, bananas for a 'healthy' snack, were feeding the Candida which was giving me chronic fatigue and was keeping me fat. Once I learned from Judy's intuitive techniques about what to eat for my body's optimum health, I quickly lost kilos of weight and kept it off.

When I moved to Toronto, Canada, I put on nearly two stone. I was busy and got sucked into eating 'healthy' fast food again, like baked potatoes and brown bread sandwiches. Then I decided, out of curiosity, to be tested for food sensitivities, this time using Electro-Dermal Screening. The results exactly matched Judy's. I went back to avoiding lots of 'healthy' foods that weren't at all healthy for me and lost a lot of weight again.

I am now IN CONTROL of my weight. You can't imagine what this feels like. I never thought it would happen to me. I swear to you that it's more important to me than winning a million dollars in the lottery. If I won a million dollars, I'd still be fat and therefore deeply unhappy. A million dollars can't give you willpower and it can't take away the cravings for chocolate and ice-cream. Eating right for your type almost takes willpower out of the weight loss equation. If you eat what is right for you, you stop craving chocolate, sugar and all the other things which it seemed impossible to give up. You really don't feel like eating them any more. If I do, I know I've been eating too much wheat. I just stop eating the wheat and the chocolate cravings subside. Freedom!

Meeting Judy changed my life. I'm no longer horrified by my own reflection. I look and feel wonderful. She literally freed me from life in a fat-suit. Fat wasn't what I was meant to be in, even though I'd been fat since I was a baby. She made it really easy to keep the weight off; much easier and healthier than any diet on the market today. Thank you Judy from the bottom of my heart.
Penny Montford

THE BODY TALKS...

THE TRUTH ABOUT FOOD AND EATING FOR LIFE

What if you could talk to the body and ask it anything you wanted.........

...And it knew the answer to every question, whether it was physical, biological, mental, emotional or spiritual...

...And it knew how to cure itself and had a direct access to a universal all-knowing consciousness...

...And it had a complete memory of every event, health condition or trauma

How amazing would that be

Well it appears we can do just that.

Welcome to my incredible journey into the world of food.

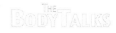

Case History: Inflammatory Bowel Disease
Amal, Age 14, Blood group B

Amal had been diagnosed with Inflammatory Bowel Disease (IBD) by specialists four years previous to consulting me in October 2001. He was very sick with severe abdominal pain and bleeding in his stools. He had swollen painful joints, particularly in his knees. He had recently spent 5 weeks in hospital with one leg in plaster, on high antibiotics to try and stabilize the deterioration. Doctors had put him on high doses of steroids and immuno-supressants to control the symptoms for the four years and any attempt to take him off them had been unsuccessful. I had never been confronted with such a serious case in a young boy. IBD is categorized medically as an auto-immune disease with unknown pathology and no known cure.

His body revealed to me his symptoms were caused entirely by severe food intolerances, verging on allergy which attacked the membranes lining his digestive system and his joints. These were wheat, soya, corn, yeast, chicken, shellfish, all citrus fruit, grapes, onions, tomatoes, olives, peanuts, pistachios, sunflower seeds and coffee. His adrenal gland function was only 22% (above 65% is healthy on my scale) and 90% of the surface area of his gut was badly inflamed. His thyroid was hyperactive by 15% and his pituitary gland only functioned at 60% of its optimum due to the effects of the steroids on his body. These are my figures which the body gives me and were not medical tests.

Amal found it difficult to be very strict on the diet but made enough changes to begin to see some improvement. After reading him the riot act a couple of times he made a huge effort to be strict and by August that year we began to see a dramatic improvement. His body confirmed that the inflammation had healed 85%, confirmed by medical blood tests that also indicated a huge improvement. His adrenal gland immune system function was still struggling, due to the continued use of the auto-immune suppressant (AIS) and mandatory steroids. The body repeatedly requested we stop the AIS in order to free the immune system so it could heal the damage. The body denied the theory that this was ever an immune system disorder where the body for some unknown reason suddenly attacks itself, and confirmed it as a genetic and albeit serious reaction to foods particular to his individual make up. A little similar to my MS but in a different part of his body. His parents decided to give it a try and stop the AIS. He began to make a rapid recovery and his adrenal gland function leapt from the initial 22% to 85% in 2 months.

In April 2003, he began to very slowly reduce the steroids as well and when I saw him again in September 2003 he had been completely off all medication for a month with no symptoms returning. In the last 6 months he has remained healthy but does get episodes of pain if he cheats too much. He has admitted to cheating a little throughout the programme which has made his progress much slower than I would have expected, but he now has the disease in hand and throughout his life will be able to manage it completely through his diet.

CHAPTER 1

STOP ALL THIS DIET NONSENSE.
DIETS DON'T WORK...

Most of the established rules of weight loss you are familiar with are actually dangerous for your health. A low calorie, low fat, high exercise programme starves your body of vital nutrients and damages your delicate immune system, ensuring that your body will just get sicker. Weight loss is a healing issue, not a fat loss issue. Excess weight is an outer sign that your body has not been getting the right balance of nutrients for your individual body type, lifestyle and exercise levels, and that your delicate hormonal system and organ functions have become damaged in some way.

The two most precious possessions you have in your life are wired into your body. They are your immune system and your metabolic rate, and they are entirely your responsibility. Both of these are influenced constantly by which foods you choose to eat, when you eat them, how you eat them, all combined with your lifestyle.

The immune system and the metabolic rate are the foundations of weight control and to a great extent your health. Without your health, nothing else matters. If your immune system drops below 75% of its optimal function, your health and well-being are increasingly at risk. If your metabolic rate drops, your body's ability to burn off calories, use nutrition, and function in its myriad of intricate systems, is compromised.

Over time your body has become toxic with an accumulation of food intolerances, chemicals, excess sugar and toxins created by incomplete digestion. Unless you first heal your body at a deep cellular level, diets and aggressive exercise aggravate the problems and leave you stripped of vital nutrients, tissue and muscle mass. Your glands, immune system and organ function are put under more stress and subsequently less efficent leaving you even more prone to weight gain. Hence the yo-yo effect of dieting. It is vital that your body receives enough calories, protein, fats and nutrients daily to heal itself and remain healthy and energetic. The efficiency with which your body digests, absorbs and uses these nutrients and calories is a function of many complex systems and glands in your body. Excess sugar and carbohydrates, food intolerances, chemicals, smoking, prescription drugs, pollutants, stress, low

Case History: Overweight, High blood pressure, Cholesterol
Ralph, age 54, Blood group A+

When Ralph came to see me in November 2001, he was taking drugs for his high blood pressure, had an irregular heartbeat, backache and was very overweight. I found his system was overloaded with food intolerances, which were affecting his adrenal and thyroid glands. Within one month of avoiding his intolerances, typical to the A blood type intolerance pattern listed in the book, he had lost an amazing 8kg and was feeling wonderful. He continued to lose the weight on the programme and has found it so beneficial that he has stuck to this way of eating ever since. Within 6 months his blood pressure and cholesterol normalized and his back ache completely disappeared. When I spoke to him in January 2004, he was still feeling and looking great.

Case History: Eczema
Tom, age 35, Blood group O-

Tom first came to see me in March 2002. He had been suffering with eczema and dry skin for many years and had recently developed psoriasis on his scalp. His body showed the problems to be 50% food intolerances, mainly wheat and 50% build-up of pesticides in his system which his genetic make up could not detoxify or tolerate as they accumulated. He commented that the psoriasis type skin condition had only started following a fruit and vegetable week detox programme he had done 5 months previously. It was clear that the concentration of pesticides eaten over that week had pushed his tolerance level into the red band. Without specific avoidance of pesticides and certain supplements to draw out the toxins, the symptoms were becoming permanent. He avoided his food intolerances, ate as much organic food as possible and took three months of Vitamins A, C and B12, Pycnogenol, Pantothenic acid and the herbs Cascara Sagrada and Sasparilla, as prescribed by his body. Within 3 months all his symptoms disappeared. Two years later he is still well but notices a return of his eczema if he indulges in his food intolerances too frequently.

calorie and low fat diets, alcohol and stimulant abuse damage these.

When I look at the 'The Body Talks' programme in its entirety, now that most of the pieces are in place, the body has prescribed itself an amazingly balanced programme based on common sense.
It is simply natural.

Its basic premise is a return to nature's original foods, eaten often, as fresh as possible, in their natural form, and cooked well and simply.

The body's rules include eating a balanced regular diet of three meals consisting of proteins, carbohydrates and fats at every meal, recognising and eliminating the impact of food intolerances, not exercising too much in the early days of a weight loss programme, cutting right down on starch and complex carbohydrates for the first few months of the programme and ensuring your calorie intake measures no less than 1700 calories a day.

Perhaps for many, the most surprising of these rules is the restriction of exercise in the early days of weight loss. Most people's immune system is just not strong enough to undergo an exercise programme beyond a moderately active 30 minute walk 4 times a week. Exercise when your immune function is low and it just serves to damage the system further. Once your system has started to heal however, you will have the energy and vitality to start exercising, as well as the health to get the real benefits from it.

The Body Talks programme is not just another diet. It is the culmination of six years of conversations with your bodies. It is a life programme of balanced healthy eating. It will change many of your preconceptions of dieting and healthy eating. It will reinforce many too.

Without fail, after following this balanced simple natural programme as prescribed by their bodies, people reported not only great weight loss but also other benefits: particularly in mental and emotional well-being. As the brain received the correct nutrients for balanced brain chemistry and was no longer adversely affected by food intolerances, people reported feeling more serene, more able to cope with stress, less aggressive and more patient. Emotional problems shrank from mountains back into molehills.

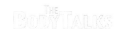

A good lifestyle programme must be realistic in our modern lifestyles; simple, sustainable, affordable, long-term and effective. Ultimately, unless we realise that our modern diets are unsustainable, that chemicals are poisoning us and our bodies cannot resist a lifetime onslaught of increasingly refined unnatural foods and current day over-indulgence, we will never be healthy for long. At some point, and I hope it is not when you have already lost your health, you will recognise that eating well for life with only the occasional indulgence is no longer a choice. With the growing threat of super bugs and viruses, the pressure from advertising to eat "new" Frankenstein foods and the stress and burden of the modern lifestyle, your immune system may be the only protection between you and a lifetime of ill health. Protect yourself with everything you have. A complete holistic approach and the adaptation to a new way of eating for life is the only way to achieve a long lasting, healthy and beautiful body.

It is interesting to observe that all of nature's foods that man has lived well on for the last hundred thousand years have been systematically lambasted in the last fifty years. This has corresponded with the development of new man-made foods by the rising food manufacturing companies, which provide more of the finance for these studies, and whose bottom line is profit and loss. The huge sales achieved by 'proving' scientifically that their man-made foods are somehow better than natures', have more than justified millions of dollars being poured into research programmes which have fortunately always come out in their favour. Become a smart consumer, do not fall for any marketing that benefits a big manufacturer. It is not necessarily unbiased.

If we do not wake up (within the next 10 to 20 years) and smell the roses quickly, truly good food may simply just not be available without genetic modification, adaptation or high chemical residues. Support good farming practices whenever you can, trust that nature really does know best and, if in doubt, ask how much man has been involved in the food you are about to eat!

Sustainable weight loss must ensure that a deep healing process takes place and that actual weight loss is very slow. The normal pattern of weight loss on The Body Talks Programme is very different from one you expect and purposely much slower. However, the change in your volume, vitality and well being more than make up for the longed for rapid loss on the 'God of Scales'. You will replace pound of fat for pound of muscle until your genetic muscle mass has been rebuilt, but as fat has much more volume than muscle, you will shrink in volume, though the scales initially will not reflect this. Many of my clients on the programme looked like they had lost a couple of stone and felt fantastic. They are toned and much smaller. But the scales have not budged a millimetre. So frustrating!! Not really.... Once your muscle mass is rebuilt your metabolic rate will jump and then you will slowly burn off that stubborn fat.

Throw away your preconceptions of dieting and your scales. They indicate nothing. A healthy slim person should be heavy for their height if their body muscle mass percentage is high and their body fat index is low. Remember, muscle is two and a half times heavier than fat. I have found time and time again that when the body says it is at its ideal weight for optimum health, the client is still adamant that they need to lose a further 3kgs on average. The body however, strongly disagrees and the fight to lose these last few kilos is fought very strenuously by the body. Our ideal is culturally based on the concept of carrying absolutely no fat whatsoever, a level generally considered too low for good health.

Because this eating programme is balanced, it allows the body to find its ideal weight over time, whether this means losing weight or putting it on. The optimum nutrition intake feeds your body with vital nutrition without putting on fat, which particularly appeals to anyone suffering with anorexia or bulimia. I have had three very successful cases of young women overcoming long-term eating disorders using the Body Talks Programme. By eating small balanced meals little and often, they laid down muscle and not fat and were slowly able to build up their confidence in food again. It is however, vital that anyone suffering with an eating disorder also receive counselling and support from a professional therapist.

Case History: Irritable Bowel Syndrome
Female, British, age 35, Blood group O

I was 3 stone overweight between the birth of my two children who are now 6 and 9 years old. I tried every type of diet available with only moderate success. Then I started having symptoms of IBS and simply dreaded being invited out for a meal in anticipation of the effects. The IBS became progressively worse and I was admitted to hospital twice with infected blockages in my colon. Eventually I had a colonoscopy and although the specialist detected that something was definitely 'not right', no cure could be found. I resorted to taking antispasmodic medication and peppermint oil, which alleviated my suffering a little.

Having followed the medical route to eliminate any more serious complications, I felt my next step was to contact Judy. I had been given Judy's number a while ago but wanted to have myself checked out medically first.

My first visit to Judy in June 2002 was a revelation. I followed the advice given, and by day 5 the detox hit me! I felt dreadful and my body was covered with boils! However, by the end of the second week I started to feel much better and even started losing weight. Six months later I have lost a staggering 16 lbs. Friends who haven't seen me for a year simply cannot believe I am the same person. My IBS symptoms have gone, although I have to be very careful to avoid my intolerances as I have had quite severe reactions to small amounts of the 'wrong' foods. I now look and feel healthier than I have for many years. I'm full of energy and am constantly amazed that I can have plenty to eat and am still losing weight.

THE BODY TALKS PROGRAMME IS BASED ON THE FOLLOWING UNDERLYING PREMISES:

- The healing of the adrenal and endocrine glands by relieving them of the constant burden of food intolerances.
- Triggering detoxification of accumulated food intolerance and chemical residues stored in the body cells, which put an increasing strain on all the body's functions, particularly the liver.
- The re-laying down of muscle mass through correct regular consumption of protein, so increasing metabolic rate which will in turn burn off more calories and excess fat.
- NOT undertaking strenuous exercise for the first stage of the programme to give the immune system a chance to heal. The protein you are trying to lay down as new muscle will just be used to exercise the current muscle. Exercise is gradually increased to an ideal level of 40 minutes of moderate aerobic activity, four times a week, combined with stretching, or one or two yoga classes. A more intensive exercise programme must not be undertaken until the system is healed, indicated by a deep feeling of well-being.
- Learning to eat the correct ratio of proteins, carbohydrates and fats at each meal. This correct ratio ensures that the body receives all the nutrients it needs for the next three to four hours without laying down excess calories as fat. A balance of these foods at each meal also triggers the optimal balance of hormones and brain chemicals.
- Ensuring adequate calorie intake to stimulate increased metabolic rate.
- The use of particular vitamins and minerals to boost the immune system, balance brain chemistry, help with cravings and repair struggling organ function.

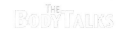

I do not give a daily menu on this diet. I feel it is vital that you understand foods and the rules of good eating so you can adapt your own diet to your own preferences and lifestyle. I cannot tell you to eat chicken on a Tuesday: your body may want fish. Many of the recipes given in diet books that you are supposed to follow strictly for the duration of the programme take time and planning, that most people just don't have. As a result, instead of understanding why we are eating something, we follow the programme without thinking and then when we find it too difficult, drop off it. These programmes also fail to teach us about a way of eating for life. During the last year my clients have come from every corner and culture in the world. The rules for good balanced eating are the same, but food preferences differ hugely from each other, whether you are Asian, Arabic, Oriental, Western, South American or African.

Learn about food and then you will know how to eat well in any culture.
The rules are simple and can be followed easily within the confines of eating out, travelling and eating on the run.

Much as I would like to tell you to always sit down to eat, chew properly and enjoy your food, eat well when travelling and never cheat, it is just not realistic in modern day life. At least if you can understand what you are eating, or the extent to which you are cheating, you will be able to repair it and your body will balance out in the long run.

Good Luck!

CHAPTER 2

FOOD INTOLERANCES

Without the right balance of nutrients for your individual body type, lifestyle and exercise levels, it is very likely that your delicate endocrine system, metabolism and organs are not functioning in their optimum state. A lifetime of eating foods that are not suited to your body type can lead to all manner of conditions - most commonly, weight gain.

In order to redress the body's balance, and to assist as it heals itself, you must understand how to eliminate the toxins that have accumulated in your system. Following a deep cellular detox, you will be guided towards balanced eating practices and shown how and why we really get fat.

Having listened to over 2000 bodies, I have discovered that food intolerances play a major part in holding us back from health. Approximately 80% of my patients have seen significant improvements simply by avoiding foods to which their bodies are intolerant.

Unless we eliminate certain foods, we are subjecting our bodies to systematic assault from toxins particular to our personal genetic makeup. Without an elimination of food intolerances, it is impossible to truly heal the body as they place a constant and increasingly intolerable burden on our systems.

What do food intolerances do to the body?

Depending on your blood type and cultural inheritances, and as a result of the dramatic changes that have been made to our foods during the course of the past century, your body will react to some foods as though they are attacking it.

This reaction will trigger your immune system to release antibodies, and over time this will exhaust your vital immune controlling glands situated above the kidneys, called the Adrenals. If these glands become weak, they affect the function of every other endocrine gland in the body. Your digestive system is also under attack as it will not be able to properly digest these foods, leaving residues stored in the body's cells. When this level reaches saturation point, these toxic residues spill into the bloodstream in levels greater than the body can clear, causing a decline in the body's health.

Headaches, sinus problems, acne, fatigue, hormonal imbalances, digestive problems and even arthritis and allergies can be caused in this way. Although it may seem very sudden, the condition will have been slowly developing in the body, eventually reaching a critical level, at which point symptoms are suddenly exhibited.

You will not even have been aware that your immune system has struggled to fight invaders every single time you ate foods that were not suited to your body. It's time to call a cease-fire and give your overburdened immune system a well-earned rest!

Identifying food intolerances and strictly eliminating them from your diet for an initial period of two months is a vital first step to healing your body. Avoiding foods you are intolerant to will give your body an opportunity to rid itself of built up toxins, and allow the healing process to begin. I now strongly believe that no long term weight loss programme can be truly successful until food intolerances are recognised and eaten only occasionally over a lifetime.

Which foods should I avoid?

In his excellent book, 'Eat Right 4 Your Type', Dr Peter D'Adamo identifies a wide range of foods that should be avoided according to blood type. Besides Dr D'Adamo's pioneering work in this field, my experience with more than 2000 clients from many different cultural backgrounds, must rate as one of the most extensive independent studies done in the world to date. It is based on multiple case studies and inferences that have been co-related and researched over several years for tangible and verifiable results. Dr D'Adamo's best selling book detailed both his and his father's work over 40 years into the biological impact of different foods on different blood types. Their findings on how different foods affect the health and weight of different blood types and the history of the evolution of man and food through the ages, make a lot of sense. Thousands of people have felt the benefit of following his recommendations. In many ways The Body Talks is both an endorsement and development of their work.

In my own practice, I have developed a very accurate ability to test food intolerances through asking the body via muscle testing, and, according to the body, have found that the list of food intolerances can be actually far less restrictive for everyday living than Dr D'Adamo's research indicates. Even if many of these foods do appear to have an effect on the blood, the body says it is actually able to deal with many of them due to the fact they are either not being eaten often enough to build up to a critical level or the body has another ability to detox them that we do not yet know about. My question to the body when testing for intolerances is, 'Which foods are damaging your health?' My opinion is that by following his recommendations too closely, many foods that are actually quite nutritious are being unnecessarily avoided, when they are not actually doing any real harm. The body has also advised against giving people the foods that are highly beneficial for them as the tendency is to eat an excess of them at the expense of a diet with more variety and balance.

In addition to this my experience strongly indicates that the biological relationship between the body and diet is not fully explained by blood testing for food intolerances. Nine times out of ten I am able to guess people's blood type correctly thanks to Dr D'Adamo's guidelines, which confirmed my initial observation of four distinct patterns similar to his. Until his book came out I had not linked the patterns so closely to blood types. Observation of the healing of conditions caused by food intolerances has now led me to believe we are still missing something and that food intolerances may not always register a reaction in blood tests, but may directly impact the gut, the brain, the endocrine glands or the joints on an individual genetically determined basis. At this stage I believe that only the individual body can tell us what it cannot tolerate and the reasons for this, through Kinesiology or Vega testing, which relies on electrical impulses in the energy field. Science has yet to develop a fully accurate way of assessing them. If I get a client in who is experiencing several different symptoms such as irritable bowel problems, headaches and a skin rash which the body confirms are all due to food intolerance as opposed to other factors, I can then ask the body exactly which foods cause which symptom. Not all foods attack the same parts of the body. The IBS may be caused by wheat and coffee, for example, whereas the headaches might be a reaction to lettuce and the skin rash a different reaction to oranges. Only the body can tell us this, I doubt there will ever be a blood test that will be able to pinpoint this relationship to this accuracy.

I am naturally biased to Kinesiology as a testing method, but it does rely to some extent on the skill of the practitioner. The Vega test is the next most accurate as it also works with the electrical bio frequencies on the atomic level by registering the electrical responses of the body to certain foods. The most available and well known test for intolerances is a blood test called the Nutron test, where the foods are introduced to the blood one by one and the level of the response of the immune system is measured. I have seen more than 80 clients who have had a food intolerance blood test done, and then come to me for re-testing. In every case the results have differed significantly from my testing, but my testing got the long term results and alleviation of symptoms, even though the Nutron recommendations had been followed strictly for several months. I myself had the test done in 1991, before I was diagnosed with Multiple Sclerosis and, if I had followed its advice, would be in a wheelchair today. My test did not reveal an intolerance to chicken, which was the main cause of my Multiple Sclerosis, something I know for sure as I go numb in my left big toe if I eat chicken more than twice in a period of seven to ten days.

So I am left with the onerous burden of trying to give you a realistic but effective guideline of foods that I think you will most likely be intolerant to according to your blood type. These foods must also be eaten regularly enough in most people's diets, to qualify as worth giving up for a period of time to bring about a worthwhile change.

As it is impossible to provide a completely accurate list of all intolerances without undertaking individual muscle testing, I have repeatedly observed the following foods as the most significant common intolerances for each blood group and this list can be relied upon as a good starting point for your detox programme.

There are four main blood groups. 'O', 'A', 'B' and 'AB'. Each of these can be either positive or negative but this is not relevant to your food intolerances. I have observed that the negatives of each blood type do appear to have fewer strange intolerances than the positives but that the ones that they do have, such as those named over the page, appear to be more vicious.

You will need to find a clinic to test your blood-type before you begin this programme unless you already know it. Probably as many as seventy percent of people do not know their blood type when they come in to see me.

Feeding Children!

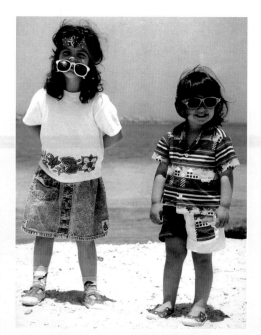

I treat many children of all ages from as young as a few months old, particularly with eczema and tummy troubles. Food intolerances are apparent from birth and can be given to the infant through the mothers' milk. This can be a problem if the mother is one blood type and the child another but when the mother has done her best to avoid her babies intolerances, they have found that colic and sleep improves.

It is important not to take children off their possible intolerances too strictly but to give their bodies a chance to taste and digest every possible food that they may come across as adults. Unless the food may be directly causing a skin condition, Attention Deficit, hyperactivity or other behavioral problem, which can only be known through individual testing or lengthy elimination diets, reduce the intake of the foods that are listed under their blood type. You must ensure they eat a little of them each week. In this way their taste buds and digestive systems become accustomed to a wider variety of foods but any build up of residue from a particular food is kept to a minimum.

Children must be fed a balanced nutritious diet following all the rules of this programme for ultimate health, which includes a little protein at every meal, plenty of natural fats, limited sugar and wholesome starches. Eggs are excellent for children and I have been horrified to hear of parents keeping theirs off eggs in case of high cholesterol. The yolk of an egg is the best brain food available to any child. Many foods such as fish and some vegetables are toxic to young tummies and if your child objects strongly to a food on more than three offerings do not force feed it. It is likely due to them instinctively knowing it is not good for them. It takes about three tastings for a child to develop a liking for a new food and if a child rejects a food at any meal, do not push it and create a scene. Children learn through example and will watch you enjoying it. Gently reintroduce the food again a few months later and see whether the taste has developed yet.

A final word of caution. Your attitude to food and eating will influence your child through-out their life. The emphasis should be on regular healthy balanced meals, enjoyment of all foods at appropriate times, appreciation that everyone has their own likes and dislikes without forcing them to eat anything, education about and the strict limitation of junk and fast foods and a generally relaxed fun approach to meals and food. Please do not make a big thing about your child being overweight, particularly with girls and the impossible pressure to be thin. Girls develop a healthier hormonal system for life if they are carrying a little puppy fat at puberty and any fad diets at this age can be very damaging. As long as children are educated about food and eating a balanced diet, they will naturally grow out of any excess in their teens. Encourage regular exercise. Beware of allowing excessive use of toiletries, deodorants and cosmetics which all contain unnecessary chemicals. Be an example and use natural detergents and body products.

Case History: Insomnia
Katherine Gardner, age 9, Blood group A

"I still can't get to sleep" was the constant cry from Katherine, two hours after she'd gone to bed. She would also wake-up during the night and just lay there wide awake. We hoped she would eventually grow out of this pattern. Judy diagnosed food as the only cause of her insomnia, namely wheat, tomatoes and of all things, lettuce. Judy said lettuce is often a cause in many insomniacs and it may account for the old wives recommendation not to eat salad at night. Upon following Judy's dietary advice, I was amazed when the following night Katherine went to bed at her usual time having eaten none of the offending foods that day – not to be seen again until the next morning. She slept soundly and without waking once and this is now the normal pattern. We are amazed and delighted by such an instant result. To prove the point, should she unavoidably cheat at a birthday party or eat something mistakenly, she immediately pays for it with a disturbed sleep that night.

O Blood Type

Characteristics of the O Blood type
More than 50,000 years old
The original 'hunter-gatherer'
Strong, hardy digestive tract
Thrives on physical exertion and regular exercise
Needs red meat in diet to strengthen immune system

Foods to avoid include:
- Wheat
- Lactose in milk (60% of O types are lactose intolerant, so use your instinct to guide you: if you don't like milk, avoid it!)
- Full milk cheeses, such as cheddar, edam, cream cheese, cottage cheese (No need to eliminate butter, yoghurt, or high protein cheeses such as feta, mozzarella, halloumi and goat's cheese)
- Soya (unless you have South East Asian or South American heritage)
- Oranges
- Tomatoes
- Shellfish (crab, lobster, prawns, oysters, mussels, calamari)
- Peanuts and pistachios
- Tea (Indian and Chinese black tea such as breakfast tea and Earl Grey)
- Coffee (in all forms, including decaffeinated)
- Hot spices (e.g. curry, chilli, pepper, paprika) You may eat them mild and in moderation.
- Mono Sodium Glutamate (found in Chinese food and processed meats)

All blood types should endeavour to eliminate all chemicals such as artificial sweeteners, Monosodium Glutamate, the chemical flavour enhancer found particularly in Chinese food and processed meats and smoked meats.

Case History: Knee Pain
Male, age 42, Blood group O

I came to see Judy about a year and half ago with knee problems. It was to a point that I remember having difficulties crossing my legs without pain for more than 10 seconds. Going up the stairs I could hear my knees cracking.

I was previously told that nothing was wrong either with my ligaments or with my muscles or my joints. Nobody could tell what was wrong.

Judy told me I was intolerant mainly to wheat, coffee and tea.
The cure was as simple as changing my diet, which I did without any difficulties. I even actually enjoyed trying new products I never looked at before.

I could feel it really improving after a couple of months and it's now totally cured, without any medication, just by watching what I eat. My immune system is now around 82 to 85% and I really feel in good health. I have not suffered from a cold since I started the programme.

Just as an anecdote, Judy diagnosed the intolerance in June 2001. In October 2001 I was climbing Mount Kilimanjaro-not without difficulties: the altitude was giving me trouble, not my knees!
I just wanted to say thank you.

Vincent Gall

A Blood Type

Characteristics of the A Blood type
Around 10,000 B.C
First cultivators of grains and livestock
Sensitive digestive tract
Tolerant immune system
More resistant to virus
More prone to heart disease, cancer and diabetes

Foods to avoid include:
- Wheat
- Lactose in milk
- Full milk cheeses, such as cheddar, edam, cream cheese, cottage cheese (no need to eliminate butter, yoghurt, or high protein cheeses such as feta, mozzarella, halloumi and goats cheese)
- Soya (unless you have South East Asian or South American heritage)
- Red meat (pork, lamb, beef and veal)
- Tropical fruits (including bananas, dates, figs, mango, guava, papaya, kiwi, watermelon, passion fruit)
- Tomatoes
- Monosodium Glutamate (found in Chinese food and processed meats)

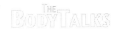

Case History: Back Pain
Sherry, 37 years old, Blood group A

Sherry came to see me because she had a slipped disc on L5 that was touching the spinal cord. Her back problems had been chronic for many years, but had become acute in the past four months. The pain was excruciating, radiating down both legs and even the most powerful painkillers provided little relief. Sherry was scheduled to have a back operation four days after her consultation with me.

Sherry's body told me that the pain was not the result of a slipped disc, but of severe inflammation in the spine caused by a build up of food intolerances, particularly dairy products and tropical fruits. Sherry said that she had been eating fruit, particularly her favourites, such as bananas and mangoes, every morning.

More than willing to postpone the operation in favour of the diet I recommended, Sherry found that just two weeks after eliminating her food intolerances, the pain was less severe and movement was much easier. Two months later, Sherry suffered only mild pain that was relieved completely by undertaking special gym exercises four times a week.

Five months later, Sherry ordered a fruit cocktail, not realising that it contained mango. Within five hours of drinking the cocktail, she was in excruciating pain again and remained flat on her back for 24 hours. The pain was relieved mostly by Ponstan (a strong anti-inflammatory), but took another two weeks to disappear completely.

Sherry is now pain-free-as long as she avoids her food intolerances-and is slowly strengthening her back after the years of inflammation have weakened her muscles. Sherry is one of many patients I have seen whose long-term back problems were a direct result of food intolerances.

B Blood Type

Characteristics of the B Blood type
Appeared around 3,500 BC
The nomad
Balanced
Good resistance to viruses
Least prone to heart disease and cancer
Most prone to immune system disorders such as MS and Lupus
Good with dairy foods

Foods to avoid include:
- Wheat
- Corn
- Chicken
- Pork
- Shellfish
- Oranges
- Soya (unless you have South East Asian or South American heritage)
- All nuts, except almonds and cashews; avoid peanuts, pistachios and sunflower seeds in particular
- Tea (Indian and Chinese black tea such as breakfast tea and Earl Grey)
- Coffee (in all forms, including decaffeinated)
- Hot spices (e.g. curry, chilli, pepper, paprika)
- Monosodium Glutamate (found in Chinese food and processed meats)

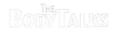

Case History: Cough and tennis Elbow
Male, British, age 50, Blood group B

I came to see Judy complaining of a constant cough. I also had tennis elbow and tingling fingers. Judy diagnosed my symptoms as the result of food intolerances with no other complications. I was initially very sceptical that just food could cause so many problems and such pain in my elbow. However, I followed the programme strictly and to my amazement saw a dramatic improvement in all my symptoms. My cough disappeared almost overnight! I also lost 7kg in weight and more than 2 years later am still feeling well.

Case History: Arthritis
Sarah, 25 years old, Blood group B

Sarah made an appointment to see me seven months after developing massive swellings in her feet, wrists and neck. She had been diagnosed with arthritis and had been prescribed strong medication for the pain and to reduce the swelling. Her sister also suffered from similar, less severe symptoms.

During her consultation, Sarah's body revealed a high genetic propensity for arthritis (60%), and also that the gene was triggered entirely by food intolerances. Sarah's adrenal function was only 43%, and she was intolerant to wheat, corn, yeast, beef, pork, chicken, shellfish, grapes, oranges, cucumber, olives, tomatoes, peanuts, sunflower seeds, tea and coffee, MSG and alcohol. Sarah's body asked for supplements of vitamin B12 and chlorophyll from green algae.

One month after eliminating her food intolerances, Sarah had improved by 80%. The swelling had gone, and the pain was less severe. Over the next few weeks, Sarah was able to come off the drugs, and suffered only occasional aching in the balls of her feet. I recently bumped into Sarah, at a Salsa class! Two years later she has made a complete recovery, but said that mild pain returns if she does not restrict her intake of those foods to which she is intolerant.

AB Blood Type

Characteristics of the AB Blood type
Only around 1000 years old
Adaptable to environmental and dietary changes
Sensitive digestive tract
Rarest blood type (2-5% of population)

The AB blood type is the most evolved having recently appeared only in the last 1000 years, and on the whole usually has very few intolerances. However, the AB can inherit any combination of intolerances from either the A, B or even both bloodtypes, making it very difficult to generalise without individual testing. However, the following lists the most common offenders in 90% of AB's I have seen. Your natural likes and dislikes are your best guide in addition to the following list. Around 40% of AB's will be fine eating milk products.

This blood type will need to avoid foods listed under A and B blood types. The specific list will vary from individual to individual, but tends to include:

- Wheat
- Lactose in milk
- Full milk cheeses, such as cheddar, edam, cream cheese, cottage cheese (No need to eliminate butter, yoghurt, or high protein cheeses such as feta, mozzarella, halloumi and goat's cheese)
- Chicken
- Oranges
- Soya (unless you have South East Asia or South American heritage)
- Monosodium Glutamate (found in Chinese food and processed meats)

The AB blood type is the only blood type that can fully tolerate tomatoes. The tomato was a highly poisonous fruit until around 1000 years ago, about the time this blood type first appeared. All other O, A and some B's retain a genetic memory of its acidity and toxicity.

Case History: Headaches, Back pain
Jacqui, Blood group O

I've been on the herbs and vitamins now for a little over two months and have been good (mostly) about my intolerances. The sweating has disappeared. Hooray!!! For the first time in years I'm no longer embarrassed. The headaches no longer seem to be triggered by stress but are definitely triggered by storms. I'm sleeping well (though I can't seem to sleep enough!), I have more energy, and I've lost about 6 pounds (2.5 kg) since I saw you last. My doctor noted that my blood pressure (always in the normal range) is now much lower (still in normal, but bordering on clinically low) at 90/60. My chiropractor said to me the other day "I don't know what you're doing to manage your stress, but this is definitely not the same back I first laid hands on."

Case History: Glandular Fever, Infertility
Fiona, Blood group A

I had very low energy levels and felt run down, constant colds, painful abdominal bloating and depression. Judy discovered I had been carrying a low grade Glandular Fever virus in my system for the past ten years and that I was highly intolerant to certain foods. The combination of the two had left my immune system totally exhausted. After taking a range of herbal supplements and going through the strict 2 month detox period, together with changing my diet, I am now enjoying the best health I have ever had. I have so much more energy to enjoy life and I haven't had a cold in 6 months. On a more recent visit (Jul 2002), Judy discovered I had inflamed ovaries and that this was causing irregular cycles and was the probable reason why I had been unable to get pregnant in the last few years. I took the herb, Pau D'Arco for a month and am pleased to report that I have had 3 normal 28 days cycles since then, and the discomfort I felt in the lower abdomen has now stopped. Judy also told me that my uterus was acidic due to a build up of bleach so I changed all my washing powders to natural products. I had an ultrasound scan to make sure that everything appeared to be in good working order, and the ovaries appeared fine. Then in April 2003 I fell pregnant easily and naturally.

WHERE DO I GO FROM HERE?

Do I have to eliminate these foods permanently?

You should begin your programme by strictly eliminating those foods identified for your blood type for a period of two months. This is how long it takes to empty the lifetime build-up of toxic residue currently stored in your cells.

Identifying your food intolerances is the first step to healing your system. A successful detox will relieve your immune system, enabling it to function much more effectively.

THE CELLULAR DETOX

I have observed that people go through the following pattern time and time again during a food intolerance-elimination programme and have called it a "Cellular Detox", as opposed to a digestive detox which we normally refer to when fasting or cleansing the body. Here we are detoxing the residues of foods our bodies have not properly eliminated from the blood and then have stored in the cells over many years. It takes the body at least two months to flush the accumulated food intolerance residue out of the cells, during which time you will have ups and downs of feeling great and terrible! A commitment to an initial strict avoidance of your foods for two months is a must on the long road to complete healing of your weight. If you are particularly overweight or suffer from any ailments which you notice improve when you avoid these foods, try and avoid them for four months in order to allow a deeper healing to take place in your cells. If for example food has been the cause of irritable bowel symptoms such as bloating, pain and gas, these foods will have left your gut inflamed. This damage can take as long as five months to repair before you feel completely better, though you feel a considerable improvement in the first two months. Keep in mind that food intolerances are not curable, just manageable, and if you ever resort to eating too many of the foods that cause your problem, it will just come back again.

The Detox Period

Once you have found out your blood type, begin your healing programme by eliminating ALL of the foods that are listed under your blood type. After five days of strict abstinence, the brain registers that no new 'bad' foods have come into the body and that the blood is now clear. The brain signals to the cells storing the accumulated toxins that the coast is clear to release some of the stored residues. On day six, you may wake up feeling like you have had a little run in with a double decker bus. If you have been experiencing any symptoms that have been directly caused by a food intolerance, the release of old stored toxins from the cells into the blood stream will trigger them all off again. It is not uncommon to experience any or all of the following for a day or more:

POSSIBLE SYMPTOMS OF CELLULAR DETOX

1. Deep fatigue and sleepiness, a drugged like feeling
2. 'Spaciness', emotional outbursts, moodiness and/or irritability
3. Worsening of any of your disorders
4. Cravings
5. Mild nausea
6. Headaches above the eyes (take a painkiller if unbearable)
7. Cold/flu like symptoms and sore throat, which can be followed by a loose mucous head cold that can last up to three weeks
8. Strange aches and pains which move around the body
9. Skin reactions such as acne, odd spots, cracked lips or rashes
10. Changes in the menstrual cycle such as sporadic or heavy periods, which will rebalance after three to four months

Most detoxes will be fairly mild and do not be put off by this list. It is actually a fascinating experience. However, in case you do have a severe reaction. I hope that by warning you that this is quite normal, you will not panic and rush down to your doctor! It will all pass.

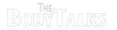

Replace your intolerances with good alternatives listed on page 42, follow the programme strictly to ensure complete detoxification as quickly as possible and ensure you maintain a balanced diet.

The first six detox symptoms will usually only last for three to four days. Then the blood clears them from the body and you will experience a period of a day or more of vitality, disappearance of your symptoms, rapid fluid loss and some weight loss. When the blood is clear again after another day or so, the next layer of residue will dump into the blood and you will feel worse again. This yo-yoing can last up to two months, with the bad times getting much shorter and less severe and the vitality periods getting longer and stronger. The other symptoms may be with you for several weeks though these will also come and go to a degree.

A rare but distressing detox symptom of avoiding your food intolerances is the development of constipation. Unbeknown to you, your food intolerance may have had a loosening affect on your bowels over many years, causing the natural bowel peristaltic movement of the small and large intestine to become lazy. When these foods are naturally eliminated, that diarrhea affect is removed and the lazy bowels may take several weeks to 3 months to begin to work normally. **Do not add fiber**. By resorting instead to softer, well cooked vegetables and fruit, the weakened bowel will slowly recover. Alow Ferox Crystals (see page 79), Psillium husks and/or senecca will aid the movement but only use these if you have no previous symptoms of irritable bowel, pain or inflammation. Drink plenty of water and be patient. The opposite affect often occurs if you have suffered with constipation before you start the elimination. Food intolerances, particularly wheat, can paralyse the gut but it quickly begins to work once the culprits are avoided.

You should try and avoid all your intolerant foods for **a minimum of two months**. You may then slowly introduce your intolerant foods very occasionally, for example only every four to five days. I would highly recommend you try and avoid wheat and dairy (if recommended for your blood type) until you have reached your ideal size and weight before introducing them back into your diet occasionally. People often report long-standing problems such as IBS and headaches, skin problems and back pain disappearing when they have eliminated their intolerances but they may need to avoid them for five or six months to allow the body to recover fully from the damage. If you are not sure what might be causing the problem, introduce one food at a time and wait 48 hours to see how it will affect you and how sensitive you are to it. If any of your symptoms return even mildly, avoid it for a further **three months** and try again. If you get no reaction, only eat that food **once every four days.**

Once you are detoxed, your delicate immune and endocrine systems then begin to heal deeply. This second stage takes up to three months on average, to repair the damage done over many years. If you cheat too often during this period, you will slowly build up the toxins again and will never reach superhealth, a feeling of incredible sustained vitality, mental clarity and strength.

This is a new science and I have not yet been able to study changes in intolerances over a long period. The body indicates to me that these are genetic and are linked to your blood type and as a result are unlikely to change during your lifetime. You will therefore always be intolerant to the foods on your list. These are not allergies and the secret is to avoid a build up of a certain food to the extent that the body can no longer cope with that amount of toxic residue. Once you have reached superhealth, you will find you can tolerate most of your bad foods occasionally without getting any serious reaction or noticing a drop in energy. It then becomes a balance, listening to your body and knowing how much or little you can get away with. I have a rule of being very strict at home and cheating only when I go out and cannot avoid it. Holidays can be repaired with two to four weeks of strict re-adherence on return, meaning life does go on!

Those who achieve even the first two months report such a renewed vigour for life that they then find it easier and easier to make this a way of life and enjoy the feeling and benefits of this lifestyle, so that they never completely go back to old ways. Commonly reported improvements include: disappearance of long term problems such as headaches, IBS, back problems, skin disorders and sinus pain; weight loss; renewed vitality, vigour and strength; and even looking and feeling much younger!

In addition to clearing your cells, the elimination of these foods will also help detoxify the liver. A healthy liver is paramount to effective weight loss and I would thoroughly recommend you undertake the liver cleanse at least once in the first two months of this programme. See chapter 11. This amazing cleanse opens up the bile glands in the liver and removes bile stones, toxins, cholesterol chaff and chemicals. It is a safe, fascinating experience to see what can actually come out of your body! Can't say its fun but it is not nearly as nasty as it sounds! ☺

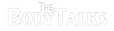

BEWARE OF........ Food intolerances are found in...

The first step to starting this programme is to familiarise yourself with foods which contain your intolerances. Here are the main ones and as you will be eating healthy natural foods this will not be difficult! However the challenge long-term comes in learning to read labels as many products may contain hidden baddies. If the food is listed near to last in the ingredients on the label, it will be present in very small amounts, which once you have completed your initial detox will not cause too much problem. That is as long as you don't eat them too often.

WHEAT:
Whole wheat flour, white flour, granary flour, bread made from any of these, pasta, bagels, pitta bread, wheat bran, pastry, couscous, semolina, wheat germ, sausages, sauces, muesli (wheat flakes), most breakfast cereals, some makes of potato chips, anything containing modified starch, cakes and biscuits.

YEAST:
Bread, vinegars, soy sauce, peanuts, anything fermented or pickled, yeast extract, (found in many foods you would not expect, check labels!) Marmite, Bovril, malt, alcohol.

Most yeasty alcoholic drinks in descending order:
(Should be avoided as much as possible for everyone for first two months)

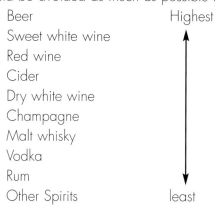

Beer	Highest
Sweet white wine	
Red wine	
Cider	
Dry white wine	
Champagne	
Malt whisky	
Vodka	
Rum	
Other Spirits	least

Why is Wheat so bad for everyone?
My experience with wheat personally and in the multitude of health problems it causes in hundreds of my clients prompts me to state that I believe modern day wheat to be responsible for many health problems today. These include diabetes, irritable bowel problems, constipation, migraines and headaches, back problems, heart attacks, strokes, allergies, ADDH and hormonal imbalances to name a few common ones. Wheat damages the immune system in around 90% of my clients and will feed many viruses if present in the body.

In the late 1860's, man began to selectively breed wheat to increase the yield of the crop. They took the original wheat grain we now call Spelt, and through cross-pollination increased the size of the germ twofold and in doing so doubled the gluten content. Modern day wheat is a completely different grain than the ancient wheat grain of our ancestors. It is also our staple diet and we eat far more than our bodies can digest and detoxify from. See A-Z for more information.

LACTOSE IN MILK:
Avoid drinking it or using it on cereals. The bacteria in <u>live</u> plain yogurt digest the lactose for you and can be eaten freely.

TOMATOES:
Apart from the obvious in salads and tomato sauces, they are used on pizza, in curry sauces, many meat sauces, sun dried tomatoes, canned soups, ketchup, tinned fish, sweet and sour sauces. Check the label or if in doubt at a restaurant, ask!

Other Substances To Avoid
Aspartame, saccharine or artificial sweeteners of any kind
Diet sodas
High fructose corn syrup
Monosodium glutamate (Chinese foods)
Wheat germ if wheat intolerant (also found in face and moisturising creams)
Genetically modified foods

SUBSTITUTE FOODS

Below is a list of the many alternatives you can eat and substitute for your intolerances. This is not a license to eat as much as you want of them, as you also need to assess what type of food they are, and how much carbohydrate, protein and fat they contain, and learn to eat them accordingly. This is clearly explained in the next chapter.

WHEAT:

- Rye crispbreads (Ryvita, Wasa)
- Spelt Flour for pastry and cakes
- Wheat free pasta
- Rice flour
- Corn flakes
- Rice Crispies
- Oat cakes
- Millet
- Maize porridge
- Rye bread
- Spelt bread   (Can be called Dinkel)
- Rice noodles
- Corn flour
- Corn thins
- Oats
- Rice cakes (refined and fattening)
- Quinoa

TEA AND COFFEE:

- Herbal teas- camomile, nettle, peppermint, fruit etc
- Green tea
- Rooibos tea or Redbush tea (from South Africa)
- Fruit juices watered down by plain or sparkling water
- $\frac{1}{3}$ juice: $\frac{2}{3}$ water

MILK:

- Goats or sheep milk/cheese
- Soya milk (only if tolerant to it)
- Rice milk (very high carbohydrate)
- Oat milk

BUTTER:
>OLIVE OIL SPREADS ONLY - no other margarines recommended.
>(Better butter recipe: mash 450g/1lb of butter with one cup of virgin olive oil, refrigerate. Gives a soft spreading butter full of good fats)

TOMATOES:
>Mango
>Tamarind (Both these make excellent sauce bases)

Case History: IBS, Hormonal Imbalance
Angie K, 33 years old, Blood group O

I had always suffered with digestion problems, namely constipation, trapped wind, heartburn, and irritable bowel symptoms. I had just learnt to live with it, but a few years ago at the age of 33, I started suffering with the dreaded 'woman' problems. I had consulted my local GP, to be told there were three options available to me, 1. HRT, 2. contraceptive pill and 3. accept it. All of which were unacceptable, but at the time decided to try option 2 which I was not happy about as I had taken the Pill for a period of 13 years when I was in my teens and stopped due to the normal health scares with any drug you take over a long period of time.

I was at my wits end, when my female colleague mentioned Judy to me. She in turn had a consultation and within one month the improvement of arthritis was amazing. As a great believer in alternative medicines, I had my first consultation back in April 2000 and was astounded by what I was told. Very high food intolerances, mainly wheat and yeast, was attributing to my digestion disorders which amazed me as I believed it to be a genetic disorder as my parents and grandparents all suffered the same. Judy is also very experienced with treating hormonal imbalances and we did start natural corrective action with Wild Yam and Agnes Castus. I adhered to the recommended Programme and was amazed at my improved energy levels, digestion and menstrual cycle.

Over the first six months, I started to listen to my body I could soon tell when I had eaten something my body doesn't like. It starts to behave and react differently, my reactions become sluggish and tattered. During this time, my mental and physical energies have improved dramatically. Just imagine where I would have been today if I hadn't found Judy, probably on HRT at the age of 37!

CHAPTER 3

ALL YOU NEED TO UNDERSTAND
ABOUT FOOD…

It constantly amazes me how few people really know their proteins from their carbs and what they really mean to their diet!! This is a must read chapter! Even though you may have read every diet book on the market and be well informed about different food groups and the unique part they play in balancing our weight and health, read through this carefully to ensure you are clear about the basics before you start the diet. The only way to ensure that you know how to choose the right foods in any situation is if you are knowledgeable about the effects of what you are eating at every meal. Unless you deeply understand the building blocks of a good diet, you will not be able to build your own programme to suit your own likes, dislikes and cultural needs. It is a bit like trying to build a great house without knowing the difference between brick and wood! Read the lists of foods carefully and the amount of nutrients they contain, so you can choose the right proportions of things just by eyeballing them and know when and what to add to balance your meals without weighing or counting anything.

UNDERSTANDING PROTEIN

I start with protein because many of you do not realise how important it is to long term health and everyday eating. Our bodies are made of protein. Every part of you, particularly the parts that reflect health and beauty, are made of protein. That firm muscle, that shiny hair, that soft silky skin, that strong bone, everything except your teeth. It is the most important nutritional element for the maintenance of good health and vitality, and is of primary importance in the growth and development of all body tissues. Proteins supply vital amino acids to the brain, which must be balanced to ensure mood stability, mental alertness, concentration and positive mind set. A protein deficiency will lead to depression and mood swings. Protein is used for the formation of hormones, which control a variety of body functions such as growth, sexual development and rate of metabolism. It also helps prevent the blood and tissues from becoming either too acid or too alkaline and helps regulate the body's water balance. It is a vital element in elimination of toxins and chemicals and a protein free cleansing programme is therefore self defeating. The word protein is derived from the Greek word meaning 'to be in first place' recognising the early brilliance of Greek physicians' appreciation of this vital food as a fundamental building block of health and perhaps the need for protein for athletic prowess!

The units from which a protein molecule is constructed are called amino acids. There are twenty two amino acids which the body uses in thousands of different combinations to build different types of protein molecules.

Amino acids are broken down into Essential and Non-essential groups. Essential amino acids must be provided in our food and there are nine of these. All the other thirteen are produced in the adult body by the liver. **High quality proteins** are foods which contain all the essential amino acids in sufficient quantity to support the growth of new tissue and balance your brain chemistry. These are what you need and they include all proteins of animal origin except gelatine, such as **meat, fish, poultry, eggs and cheese**. If just one essential amino acid is low or missing, even temporarily, protein synthesis will be reduced to the same proportion as the amino acid that is low or missing. i.e. nothing in some cases! In less complete proteins, also known as **low quality proteins**, one or more of the essential amino acids is missing. Pulses and legumes such as **lentils and beans** are rated nearly as high as animal proteins but lack or have low amounts of one or more of these essential nine amino acids. When these are combined with other foods such as **nuts, seeds and grains** which contain the proteins that are lacking in the legumes, they complement each other and provide all the essential acids to the body. If you are vegetarian it is vital therefore that you are aware of this and endeavour to combine the correct foods to ensure complete proteins. For example, legumes or pulses with either brown rice, barley, corn or sesame seeds.

There is constant renewal of all the body's cells but the rate of renewal varies greatly between different tissues. The cells of the intestinal tract are replaced every few days with new cells, the blood every one hundred and twenty days and the brain rarely. The average adult male loses approximately 40 to 60 grams of protein each day and this must be replaced by the diet. The body has no means of storing amino acids beyond a small reserve which will last for a few hours.

You must therefore try and ensure that you eat some complete protein at each meal, particularly breakfast, as you have gone around twelve hours without protein since dinner the night before. If no protein is supplied in the diet, the body will continue to break down non-vital proteins to supply amino acids to the vital body functions. Most of this will come from the muscles. If your diet is deficient in protein for a sustained period of time, you will in effect cannibalise yourself to meet your body's metabolic needs, resulting in deficient muscle mass, lowered metabolic rate, well being, vitality and strength.

> **Your body is breaking down and building up new cells, muscle, bones and tissue every minute of every day. If you do not feed your body sufficient protein to rebuild these tissues your body will have no option but to borrow protein from your muscles to replace the lost tissue in your bones and cells. You are in effect, consuming your body from the inside if you do not eat enough protein!**

On average, studies have shown that the 60% of the western population lose 40% of their muscle mass by the age of 60! This is entirely due to insufficient protein in the diet over a lifetime. If you are 40% deficient in protein you have a high deficiency in muscle mass, and the more muscle mass you have in your body, the higher your metabolic rate, the more calories you burn off, the more sugar you use, the less fat you store, the more you can eat. Keeping your muscle mass topped up is a priority. A low protein diet over many years may also be a major contributor to the development of osteoporosis or porous bones.

The recommended protein requirements differ according to the nutritional status, body size and activity of the individual. Western government recommendations have generally advised as little as 45 grams of protein for women weighing around 60kgs and 55 grams of protein a day for men weighing around 70kgs.

Time and time again, my clients' bodies have told me they eat too little protein over a day and are muscle mass deficient. On average women have requested 80-90 grams a day and men between 100 and 110 grams a day. When they have started eating this amount, split into small amounts eaten over three meals and two snacks a day, they have thrived. Liver and blood tests have shown excellent counts after three and six months on this diet.

An Asian client of mine came to me because his cholesterol and liver counts were very high. After four months on the diet he was retested. His doctor told him: "I have never seen such perfect levels in an Asian man of your age in all my years of practice. What have you done?" The doctor could not believe that my client, an O blood type, had been eating moderate but regular amounts of protein three times a day, two eggs a day without fail and red meat four times a week. This is what his and many O blood type bodies consistently request. His previous imbalances which were evident in the blood tests taken before he began this diet had not been caused by eating too much red meat or eggs, but by an insufficiency of it combined with years of a surfeit of sugars and refined carbohydrates.

A diet which is too high in protein will cause calcium to be lost from the bones and an imbalance in the potassium level in the blood. A very low potassium level is dangerous and can badly affect the heart. It is vital that you understand that this is NOT a high protein diet. It is a regulated protein diet, where optimal moderate amounts of protein must be eaten in balance with other nutrients, at regular intervals throughout the day.

Your body will not easily let you overeat protein, unless you force feed it. When it has had enough protein, either at a meal or over a period of time, it will let you know if you are listening. You will want to stop eating what is left on your plate or you may just fancy something very light at that meal. This occurs more often during the end of stage two of the programme, when your intital protein deficiency has been replenished with good diet. Then you will need to adjust portions of protein at each meal, in response to this message from your body. This protection feedback does not happen with carbohydrates-the more you eat, the more you want!

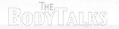

How to use the chart below

Check above to see how much actual usable protein you need to be consuming daily as a man or woman. Then go to the protein list which indicates how much absorbable protein can be utilised by the body from 1oz or 28grams of actual food eaten. For example, 1oz or 28grams, of chicken contains only about 7grams of usable amino acids for your body. A chicken breast which weighs around 5oz or 140grams provides you with 35grams of edible protein for the day. 1oz of cheese (the equivalent of one Babybel cheese) will give you 8grams of protein. An ounce of feta, a high protein, lower fat cheese, will give you around ten grams. Using this you can then eyeball how much protein you need to be consuming a day, splitting your protein needs into around 20% at breakfast, 35% at lunch and dinner and allowing the extra 10% in your snacks. Remember this is an approximation.
(1oz equals 28grams)

For example: (Excluding carbohydrates and fats.)
An average adult man needing 110 grams of protein a day could eat:

	Food	grams of usable protein
Breakfast:	2 eggs	14g
	3 rashers of bacon or turkey bacon	8g
Lunch:	168g chicken or meat	
or	50g Feta and	
	75g cold turkey	42g protein
Dinner:	168g steak or fish	42g protein
2 snacks:	10 almonds	4g
	one Babybel cheese (with one apple)	7g
	Total	**117g**

Average Adult woman

Breakfast:	2 eggs	14g
Lunch:	140g chicken or meat	
or	50g of Feta and	
	50g cold turkey cut	35g
Dinner:	140g steak or fish	35g
2 snacks	8 almonds	3g
	one Babybel cheese (with one apple)	7g
	Total	**94g**

To get an idea of how much this is, and it does not need to be exact, use the palm of your hand by about an inch thick as a guideline for the size of portion you will need at a meal. Some days you will feel the need to eat more and others less. Listen to this within reason as long as you always add some protein to each meal.

Key to colour coding

Green - Important information or eat often

Blue - Interesting information or eat in moderation

Red - Warning information or eat rarely

- Relevant information

Ounces		Grams
0.035	1	28.0
0.078	2	56.7
0.106	3	85.0
0.141	4	113.4
0.176	5	142.0
0.212	6	170.0
0.247	7	198.4
0.282	8	227.0
0.317	9	255.0

Pounds		Kilograms
2.2	1	0.454
4.4	2	0.91
6.6	3	1.36
8.8	4	1.81
11.0	5	2.27
13.0	6	2.72
15.0	7	3.18
17.6	8	3.63
19.8	9	4.08

UNDERSTANDING FOOD

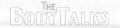

WHICH FOODS ARE PROTEINS?

ANIMAL PROTEINS 1oz of animal protein contains around 7grams of protein (1oz = 28 grams)

MEAT
Beef	Chicken
Duck	Lamb
Pork (bacon and ham)	Veal
Turkey	

FISH
Cod	Hammour
King fish	Mackerel
Salmon	Sardines
Red Snapper	Trout

EGGS   1 egg contains 7g protein

MILK (Semi-skimmed)   1 cup contains 8g protein

YOGHURT (plain)   1 cup contains 12g protein and 15 grams carbohydrate

CHEESE   1oz (28g) contains 8-10g of protein

BEST CHEESES
Cottage cheese	Cream cheese
Feta	Goats
Halloumi	Mozzarella
Ricotta	

Others:
Brie/Camembert	Cheddar
Edam	Gouda
Gruyere	Parmesan
Roquefort	Stilton

LEGUMES

Approximately ⅓ of protein to ⅔ good carbohydrates

Cooked unless otherwise noted. Each of the following portions are real carbohydrate foods containing **15gms of carbohydrate. (average cup size is 8oz).**

		Protein (grams)
Adzuki beans	¼ cup	4.3
Black beans	⅓ cup	5.0
Broad beans	½ cup	6.0
Chickpeas	⅓ cup	4.8
Black eye beans	½ cup	2.6
Kidney beans	⅓ cup	5.0
Lentils	⅓ cup	6.0
Mung beans	⅓ cup	5.0

PROTEINS THAT CONTAIN CARBOHYDRATES

NUTS AND SEEDS

Each serving contains **15 grams of Carbohydrate.** Nuts contain a lot of good fats. Nuts should be eaten in moderation as they are very high in calories.

		Protein (grams)
Almonds	23 nuts	5.8
Brazil nuts	1½ oz	5.7
Cashews	¾ oz	6.0
Coconut cream	¼ cup	2.0
Coconut milk	¼ cup	2.3
Hazelnuts	1½ oz	5.6
Peanuts	1oz	7.0
Peanut butter	2 tablespoons	8.0
Pecans	15 halves	6.0
Pine nuts	1oz	6.8
Pistachios	47 nuts	5.8
Sunflower seeds	¼ cup	8.0
Walnuts	2oz	8.2

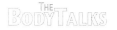

UNDERSTANDING CARBOHYDRATES

Carbohydrates are sugar! An average serving of pasta, once digested, contains the equivalent of 18 teaspoons of white sugar! A medium size apple contains the equivalent of 3 teaspoons of white sugar. A medium baked potato contains 6-7 teaspoons equivalent of white sugar in the form of starch. A head of broccoli contains 1 teaspoon of sugar. Stunning information hey?

How is that, I hear you say: potato is not sugar, bread is not sugar, they are starches? Quite right. But what few of us realise is that starch is made of thousands of simple sugars joined together. Carbohydrates are made up of three basic elements - carbon, hydrogen and oxygen. Carbohydrates can all be divided into three groups: simple sugars or monosaccharides, such as glucose, fructose and galactose; disaccharides, which are made up from two simple sugars linked together such as sucrose, lactose and maltose; and complex carbohydrates such as starch, dextrin, glycogen and fibre, which consist of thousands of simple sugars connected together. Remember, even if you are eating vegetables, you are eating carbohydrates. Because they contain complex sugar in low amounts they are considered *good* carbs and can be eaten in unlimited portions. They, more than any other form of carbohydrate, are low in sugar but provide the greatest amount of nutrients and fibre.

When carbohydrates are eaten they must be broken down by the digestive processes into simple sugars before they can be used for energy. Fibre is the exception because it passes through the body nearly unchanged as humans do not have any enzymes that are able to break it down into simple glucose.

> Therefore the main difference between a complex starch like a baked potato and a simple sugar such as an apple, is merely the time it takes the body to break the carbohydrate down into simple sugars. Complex carbohydrates, (what we know as starch), by the very fact they contain thousands of simple sugars, are a concentrated source of energy and are deceiving as to the large amount of sugar they actually provide to the body in a portion.

Once carbohydrates are broken down by the digestive process into simple sugars, they are absorbed through the wall of the small intestine into the blood and are carried to the liver. In the liver they are all changed to glucose. The glucose re-enters the blood and is then readily available as energy to the

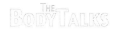

body. A small amount of glucose is changed by the liver into glycogen of which about 100 grams is stored in the liver as an emergency energy source and about 200 grams is stored in the muscles and used when they contract. Any extra sugar you eat at a meal which cannot be stored in the liver or used in the muscles is **stored as body fat!** In other words carbohydrates provide energy and little else! In fact, all refined white carbohydrates including wheat, rice, most breakfast cereals and sugar contain NOTHING else. It is all too easy to overeat sugar when eating starchy foods. A little of these is fine, but often we eat too much in one serving. Without realising it, we can easily consume 6-12 teaspoons equivalent of white sugar at one meal. If our body cannot use this energy it will turn it to body fat.

It is vital that you do not eliminate all carbohydrates from your diet. It is starches and concentrated sugars that should be eaten in strict moderation. All body functions and muscular exertion need the energy provided by carbohydrates. Fats require carbohydrates for their breakdown in the liver and to assist in the digestion and assimilation of other foods. Our brains require an average of 80 to 100 grams of sugars, including those from vegetables, a day, and anywhere from nothing to 75grams of starch, depending on size and activity levels. On average we are consuming around 150-200grams of sugar a day and 120-250grams of starch. No wonder we are battling the bulge!

Take your carbohydrates from good sources including vegetables and salads, and small amounts of whole grains. In the early stages the best of these are rye crispbreads. There are also carbohydrates in pulses, nuts, seeds, milk and yoghurt. Fruit contains concentrated amounts of a simple sugar called fructose. Do not eat too much fruit if you want to lose weight!

If we are trying to lose weight and want to use up some of the spare sugar we have stored in our bodies as body fat, we must eat less than we need so our body is forced to dip into our stores to get energy. We are over eating refined sugars and starches at such a rate, is it surprising obesity is becoming endemic?

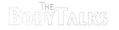

CARBOHYDRATE CONSUMPTION

The following chart is a guideline for long-term carbohydrate consumption in addition to maintaining plenty of proteins, fats, nuts, seeds, legumes and non-starchy vegetables in your diet.

Amount of Starch from refined grains, rice, bread and potato that can be eaten daily for different Body compositions

Body Composition	Stage 1	Stage 2	Stage 3
	Starch (grams) to be eaten in total per day.		
Very overweight above 8kg	0	15-30	15-30
3-8kgs overweight	0	15-30	30-60
1-3kgs overweight	15-30	30-45	30-45
Ideal weight (women)	30-45	30-45	45-75
(men)	30-45	40-50	50-80

Stage 3 depends on activity levels

EXCEPTION TO THE STARCH RULE:

Whole grain rye and spelt breads contain starch complex carbohydrate which is slow to digest, full of nutrients and good fibre and are the only exception to the starch rule. You may have ONE slice of 100% rye or spelt bread once a day in place of Rye crispbreads such as Ryvita or Wasa. These breads contain yeast and should be not be eaten at all if you are avoiding it.

In the early phase of weight loss, rely on vegetables for your carbohydrate requirements which also provide ample vitamins, minerals and fibre for proper digestion. Limit yourself to two portions of fruit a day.
As your weight returns to normal, you may begin to include more complex carbohydrates in their natural unrefined form such as brown rice, baked potato, oats and millet in addition to the slice of whole rye or spelt bread you are already allowed.

Tips to remember about Carbohydrate of all types:

- Your body does not regulate the amount of carbohydrates you eat, as it does with protein and fats. You can easily over-eat carbohydrates, leading to a greater and greater craving for them.

- Always combine carbohydrates, including fruit, with protein and fat at the same meal or within 15 minutes. If you eat fruit before a meal, do not wait more than five minutes before eating some protein. For this reason it is better to eat a main meal first and have fruit as a dessert. Contrary to eating theories of the past, particularly the Fit for Life recommendation that fruit should be eaten alone or before meals, foods do not fight and fruit does not ferment in the stomach unless you have invading bacteria in your stomach which feeds off the sugars. Fruits contain excellent raw digestive enzymes that are very beneficial in helping digestion, but this effect is lost if fruit is eaten first.

- If you are losing weight too quickly or are getting too slim; increase your carbohydrate consumption in 15g portions daily until you stop losing weight. Remember if you eat too much you will crave even more.

- To increase carbohydrate consumption only use wholegrain healthy options such as oatmeal, small baked potato, Ryvita, oatcakes, small corn on the cob, brown rice and fresh fruit.

- When you eat an excess of carbohydrates, insulin levels rise, making you hungry and tired. See the following charts on carbohydrate to see how many teaspoons equivalent of sugar you are consuming when you eat different carbohydrate foods.

CARBOHYDRATES

E.g. 1 teaspoon white sugar = 5g carbohydrate
       1 apple contains 15g carbs = 3 teaspoons white sugar!

You should be aiming to eat no more than 20 teaspoons of white sugar equivalent a day from any of the following carbohydrate sources.

E.g. 2-4 Ryvita = 3-6 teaspoons
or   1 slice rye bread = 3 teaspoons
      1-2 portions of fruit a day = 3-6 teaspoons
      1 portion starch veg = 3 teaspoons
      extra hidden carbs in yoghurt, nuts other vegetables = 5 teaspoons

TOTAL average 20 teaspoons a day

NON-STARCHY VEGETABLES - unlimited quantity

Asparagus	Cucumber	Spinach
Bamboo shoots	Eggplant	Squash
Bean sprouts	Endive	Swiss chard
Beetroot greens	Fennel	Tomatoes
Bell peppers	Garlic	Watercress
Broad beans	Green beans	Zucchini
Broccoli	Kale	
Brussels sprouts	Lettuce	
Cabbage	Lettuce - iceberg	
Carrots (raw)	Mange tout	
Cauliflower	Mushrooms	
Celeriac	Onions, Spring onions	
Celery	Parsley	
Chicory	Peppers - sweet	
Chives	Radishes	
Collards	Snow Peas	
Coriander	Shallots	

STARCHY VEGETABLES

These vegetables are chock full of good nutrients and can be eaten at any time during each stage of the programme in small portions. Avoid potato and sweet potato and count them as starch to be included later on.

Cooked. Each portion contains 15g of carbohydrate or three teaspoons of white sugar.

Acorn Squash	½ cup
Artichoke	1
Beetroot	1 cup
Butternut	⅔ cup
Carrots	1 cup
Corn	⅔ cup
Green peas	½ cup
Leeks	1 cup
Lima beans	½ cup
Okra	1 cup
Parsnips	⅔ cup
Potato (baked)	medium
Pumpkin	1 cup
Sweet potato	½ medium
Turnip	½ cup

Never peel a potato, all the goodness is packed under the skin. As soon as you peel it, it becomes nutritionless starch. Potatoes, well scrubbed and cooked in their skin, can be eaten boiled, mashed, baked or roasted.

UNDERSTANDING FOOD

FRUIT

All fruit is pure sugar! Albeit in the form of fructose, not sucrose, but still sugar and therefore still fattening. Our modern day fruit does not contain enough nutrients as most of it is picked before it is ripe and can be up to three to four weeks old before we buy it in our supermarkets. It cannot be put into a super food category and is highly over-rated as a health food, which can be eaten in unlimited amounts. Yes, it does contain digestive enzymes, making a single piece of fruit an ideal dessert after a balanced meal. But it is not a diet food. One apple contains three teaspoons of white sugar equivalent in fructose. A banana contains six teaspoons of white sugar. Eaten alone, fruit digests too quickly, resulting in too much sugar reaching the liver for it to be used immediately by the body. Any excess sugar is then stored as fat. Vegetables, however, retain their nutrient content, contain much less sugar, digest more slowly due to their higher fibre content and are a vital part of every diet. Remember fruit is also seasonal, ripening traditionally during the summer months, where it was needed to supply instant energy during the hard labour of harvesting in the summer heat of days gone by. A small amount would be stored as jam and eeked out over the long winter months, providing a little sweetness in the diet. Our annual consumption of sugar from fruit, chocolate, sweets, desserts, bread, pasta, cakes and biscuits is around 230 times more than our ancestors 200 years ago. And they worked much harder and burned off far more calories. Nutritionally they would have been less nourished from good proteins and a variety of vegetables and grains, but we are certainly overdoing the energy loading! Most bodies ask for only two 15 gram portions of fruit a day, eaten with protein or after a balanced meal. Quite simply, unless you are doing a strenuous amount of exercise, you will not be burning off more than this. Do not drink fruit juice if you want to lose weight for the same reason. It takes 4 to 5 apples to make one glass of juice…thats 12-15 teaspoons of sugar equivalent of fructose. Just because its natural does not mean it is good. It is very fattening!! If you do have them, water them right down. Beware of 'fruit only' detox diets also. They trigger huge amounts of insulin to be released and though they rest the digestion, such diets shock the rest of the body and create an imbalance in the endocrine system that takes several weeks of balanced eating to repair.

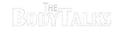

A daily intake of two portions of fruit of around 15 grams of carbohydrate each is optimum. All fruits are raw, except where noted. Each of the following natural carbohydrate portions contains 15 grams of carbohydrate.

Apple	1 small	*Lychees	7 fruit
Apples (dried)	3 rings	*Manges	½ medium
Apricots	2 medium	Melons (cantaloupe)	1 cup (cubes)
Apricots (dried)	7 halves	Melons (honeydew)	1 cup
Avocado (large)	½ fruit	Nectarines	1 medium
*Bananas	½ medium	*Papayas	½ cup (mashed)
Blackberries	¾ cup	*Passion fruit	3 fruits
Blueberries	¾ cup	Peaches	1 medium
Cherries	8 cherries	Pears	½ large
Cranberries	1 cup	Pears (dried)	1 half
Currants (dried)	2 tablespoons	Pineapple	2 slices
*Dates	2 medium	Plums	2 fruits
*Figs	2 medium	*Pomegranates	½ fruit
*Figs (dried)	1 medium	Prunes	2 prunes
Grapefruit	½ large	Pomelo	¾ cup
Grapes (large)	7 grapes	Raisins (seedless)	2 tablespoons
Grapes (small)	10 grapes	Raspberries	1 cup
*Guavas	1½ fruit	Rhubarb	7 stalks
*Kiwi fruit	1 large	Strawberries	1½ cup
Lemons	3 medium	*Watermelon	1½ cup (dice)
Limes	2 medium		

* denotes tropical fruits which should be avoided by A blood types.

GRAINS

Each of the following are starches, and the following portions contain about 15g of carbohydrate, cooked, the equivalent of three teaspoons of white sugar.

Barley	⅓ cup	Kamut	⅓ cup	Rye	¼ cup
Brown rice	⅓ cup	Millet	⅓ cup	Wheat (whole - dry)	1½ tbsp
Buckwheat	⅓ cup	Oats	⅔ cup	Wheat bran (dry)	⅓ cup
Bulgur (tabouleh)	⅓ cup	Polenta	⅓ cup	Wheat germ (dry)	⅓ cup
Corn grits	½ cup	Popcorn (popped)	2½ cups	White rice	1 tbsp
Couscous	⅓ cup	Quinoa	⅓ cup	Wild rice	¼ cup

MAN-MADE CARBOHYDRATES

You must avoid man-made carbohydrates wherever possible. Some are better than others. AVOID bread made from normal wheat. Spelt or rye is fine. The following portions contain 15 grams of carbohydrates or three teaspoons of white sugar.

Corn tortilla	1 medium	Oat bran bread	1 slice	Whole wheat bread	1 slice
Dinner roll	1 small roll	Pumpernickel bread	1 slice	Whole grain pita	1 small pita
Granary bread	1 slice	Rye bread	1 large slice		
Hamburger bun	½ bun	Spelt bread	1 large slice		

CRACKERS

Most crackers contain wheat or many additives, including hydrogenated fats. The following are acceptable and contain 15 grams of carbohydrate or three teaspoons of white sugar.

Ryvita (plain)	2 crackers	Rye wafers (Wasa)	2 crackers	Rice cakes (thin brown)	3 cakes
Ryvita (sesame)	2 crackers	Oat cakes	2 cakes		

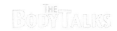

UNDERSTANDING FATS

FAT DOES NOT MAKE YOU FAT. Please get over your fear of it. When you eat fats, they do not turn into fat because they *do not stimulate insulin release*. Insulin is the catalyst needed to convert dietary fat into body fat. Fat cannot be stored in the body tissues as body fat, without the presence of sugar in the diet which triggers insulin. Insulin traps dietary fats, shoves it into fat cells and locks it in. If there is no insulin circulating in the blood stream, fats cannot be stored in fat cells.

All fats found in nature are good for you and vital for your health. Saturated, mono-saturated and polyunsaturated fats are all healthy, eaten in their natural state and in moderation. Our bodies have eaten them and evolved with them over thousands of years. Your diet should consist of 30% fats, coming from a variety of naturally occurring, unprocessed food such as olive oil, butter, eggs, red meat, avocado, poultry, fish, nuts and seeds. I cannot stress stongly enough how important good fats are for health, particularly for children.

The body needs the full range of fats found in natural foods for many vital functions in the body. The brain comprises 60% fat. Dietary fats, (as opposed to body fat already stored in fat cells), play a vital role in many different bodily functions, including metabolism, the absorption of protein and carbohydrates, the breakdown of nutrients, brain processes and the manufacture of hormones.

A deficiency of fat may result in:

- Mood disorders and depression
- Constipation
- Infertility
- Insomnia
- Sugar and carbohydrate cravings
- Brittle nails, dry skin and thin, limp hair

It takes a certain amount of fat in your meal to signal to the brain that you have eaten enough. Increase your intake of good natural fats and you will find your cravings for sugars and carbohydrates lessen. Known to be particularly important to the body and excellent at preventing heart disease are the Omega 3 and Omega 6 fatty acids. Foods containing vital Omega 3 fatty acids include fish, olive oil, nuts, seeds and avocado. Omega 6 is obtained from leafy greens, pulses and whole unrefined grains such as rye, oats and barley. Both these fatty vitamins must be consumed regularly in our food, though we are more commonly deficient in the Omega 3 fats. Omega 3 will also boost your metabolic rate and act as a diuretic.

Some people, particularly descendants of the Scandinavians, the North American coastal people and the Celtic Irish, Scottish or Welsh have a very special need for essential fats, due to their ancestors' reliance on fish for as long as 20,000 years. If you have inherited a gene from this stock, your genetic code adapted itself to a fish-based diet and you may still require lots of fish fat. Fish fats provide a very high source of the brain activating food known as DHA. People with this ancestry may not yet be able to make this out of other non-fish sources such as flax seeds, walnuts or olive oil. Without enough of this fish based Omega 3 in their diet, descendents of Scandinavians, Celts or coastal native Americans are prone to depression due to a deficiency of DHA and may find themselves craving for alcohol. If you are prone to craving alcohol to numb depression, try taking 3 capsules daily of a fish oil supplement such as cod liver oil or salmon oil and eat at least four portions of fatty fish such as salmon, mackerel, tuna or sardines a week.

Bad fats include hydrogenated fats and trans-fatty acids found in margarines, crackers, biscuits, baking and cook-in mixes, fast food, processed and packaged foods and all foods containing vegetable oils. These must be strictly limited for longterm health. The move towards vegetable oils was ill advised. A prime example of damaged man-made fats are the much processed and surprisingly fragile vegetable oils, such as canola, corn, sunflower, safflower, peanut and soya. The goodness in these oils is destroyed at the outset when they are extracted through heat. They quickly become rancid and oxidised, changing their molecular structure into indigestible and poisonous trans-fatty acids which clog your arteries and, according to talking to our bodies, also damage your brain. Extra virgin olive oil is the only exception to this rancid oil story, as the oil is cold pressed and completely natural. However, even olive oil becomes poisonous when heated. Many people have complained to me about short-term

memory loss. Shockingly, their bodies told me that the only cause of this was the effect of all heated oils when cooking. Even a little olive oil, used to fry some onions only twice a week, can, according to all the bodies I have asked including my own, be enough to damage a part of the memory in the brain and interfere with short-term memory function. All processed vegetable oils have already been heated and damaged when you buy them and even eating them cold, in salad dressings is just as damaging. They are pure poison! Only use a little butter or real ghee when frying: butter does not change its molecular structure when heated and stays stable at high temperatures. I am not suggesting you fry often anyway, but if you are making scrambled eggs or omelettes, frying a little steak or fish, or a few onions, the number of times you will need to heat fat in a week mounts up. If possible, only use butter to cook with. Use plenty of cold pressed virgin olive oil on salads and vegetables.

Processed vegetable oils are also contributing directly to unnecessary weight gain, and to some of our most common and serious health conditions, including heart disease, inflammatory and auto-immune problems such as rheumatoid arthritis, asthma and Crohn's disease, as well as osteoporosis, diabetes, colon, prostate and breast cancer. In Britain, a corn oil diet tested in 1965 actually increased the risk of dying from heart disease. Trans-fatty acids clog up our arteries. The margarine story is even worse. Our bodies cannot begin to digest and break down these man made products. It's just not natural! Eating saturated fats like butter actually increases the proportion of good cholesterol HDL's in the bloodstream. These are considered good because they take cholesterol back to the liver and are therefore thought to protect against heart disease by keeping your arteries clean. A diet low in fat and high in carbohydrates also depletes your oestrogen levels. Good oestrogen levels are needed to raise HDL cholesterol levels, the good cholesterol.

Choose semi-skimmed fat milk and dairy products and eat moderate amounts only of hard and full fat cheeses. Fully skimmed milk does not contain enough fat to stimulate the release of bile from the gall bladder, which is vital for the body to absorb calcium from milk. Do not use it!

Very good fats and foods which contain Omega 3 and essential fatty acids

Almonds
Avocado
Flax seed, sesame, walnut oil (cold pressed). Not heated
Mackerel
Olive oil (cold pressed virgin). Not heated
Salmon
Sardines
Tuna

Fats and foods which can be eaten often in moderation

Butter
Cheese
Cream
Ghee
Mayonnaise
Meat and Poultry (trimmed of fat)

Bad fats

Excess meat fat
Lard
Fried cold pressed oils including olive oil

VERY bad fats

Trans-fatty acids found in all processed oils such as corn, safflower, canola, sunflower oils, margarines, processed and fast foods, doughnuts, shop bought pastries, Chinese foods like spring rolls, fried fish, chips.
Rancid or oxidised fats
Margarines
Shortening
Buttermilk
Cream substitutes
Deep fat fried foods
Non-dairy creamers
Palm oil
Processed foods and fast foods using hydrogenated fats e.g. fries, biscuits, cakes.
Sandwich spreads

Tips to remember about Good Fats

- Real fats are vital to good health and optimum weight. Do not be afraid to eat real fats.
- Eating good fat does not make you fat. The body will only store natural fats if insulin is present in the bloodstream. E.g. pasta and cream or bread and butter. Fats eaten with proteins, vegetables and low carbohydrates will not be stored.
- A less active lifestyle does not mean that you need less fat. Nearly every process in the body involves fat and goes on at all times, regardless of your activity levels.

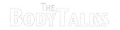

UNDERSTANDING CHOLESTEROL

The body has persistently asked for more cholesterol in its diet. I had 28 cases in the last 3 year of very high cholesterol levels in clients who had been on low cholesterol diets and/or cholesterol lowering drugs with little effect. All of their bodies asked for two eggs daily for three months, combined with a low starch, sugar and alcohol diet. When they consistently followed the body's requests and cut down on their carbohydrate and alchohol intake, amazingly they dropped to normal cholesterol levels within that period and what's more, their ratio of the bad low-density cholesterol versus the protective high-density cholesterol improved.

FATS AND CHOLESTEROL ARE GOOD FOR YOU!

Cholesterol and all types of natural fat eaten in moderation are vital to health. The fact is that in the United States, prior to 1910, people ate a diet full of saturated fats (which are notoriously high in cholesterol) and yet its rate of heart disease was much lower than it is now. Although it is high in fat, the Mediterranean diet, in which the fats are primarily mono-saturated fats from olive oil, is associated with lower heart disease risk. Greenland Eskimos, whose diet is extraordinarily high in fat, also have a low incidence of heart disease. This is now thought to be because the fat they eat comes almost entirely from cold water fish and seals, also rich in the same Omega 3 fatty acids found in olive oil, which seem to protect the heart function, despite normal cholesterol intake.

SO WHAT IS CHOLESTEROL USED FOR IN THE BODY?

Cholesterol is used as essential building material for hormones, membranes and other structures. It helps cells maintain their structure and function, and it is also the substance from which the liver manufactures bile acids, so we can digest and assimilate nutrients from food. It is essential for brain function and the stabilisation of neurotransmitters. Mood problems such as depression, agitation and irritability can occur when your body does not get sufficient cholesterol. Cholesterol also forms insulation around the nerves to keep electrical impulses moving. Without this insulation there is an increase in the potential for nerve disorders. Medical investigators at the U.S. Department of Agriculture Human Nutrition Research Centre on Ageing recently reported that cholesterol plays an important role in protecting against ageing of the brain as well as the heart. Interestingly, recent studies from the Netherlands indicate that in people older than 85 years, high blood cholesterol levels are associated with longevity and good health, owing to a lower mortality from both cancer and infectious diseases.

I have consistently found that when the body tells me that a person has a virus, the cholesterol level has been increased in order to protect the body from any damage. The cholesterol level drops back to normal once the virus has gone from the body. I suspect many inexplicable cases of high cholesterol are due to the presence of a virus in the body at the time of testing. In the case of long term chronic viral infections, the cholesterol should remain high to protect the body. Medication taken at this time to reduce cholesterol could be leaving the cells at increased danger of damage and attack by that virus. A similar reaction occurs if there is a build up of a chemical toxicity in the body, either due to an environmental polution or a genetic inability to naturally detoxify certain chemicals in everyday products. I have seen this with build ups of bleach or sodium laurate sulphate, present in many regularly used items such as cleaners, shampoos, toothpaste and body creams, which most people naturally eliminate. Families with this genetic sensitivity, may develop a responding higher cholesterol production over generations to protect the cells from damage. If this is so, as the body is strongly indicating to me, it is important that this cholesterol level be allowed to stay above normally acceptable levels to ensure that this protection is maintained.

FUNCTIONS OF CHOLESTEROL IN THE BODY

- Essential for brain function
- Makes important hormones
- Forms membranes inside cells
- Important structural building block in cell membranes
- Keeps cell membranes permeable
- Keeps moods level by stabilising neurotransmitters
- Maintains healthy immune system
- Forms insulation around nerves to keep electrical impulses moving
- Protects the body from virus or chemical damage

CHOLESTEROL AND SUGAR... WHAT HAPPENS IF I STOP EATING CHOLESTEROL?

Cholesterol is so important to your body that we all have an in-built protection should our incoming dietary levels fall below the body's vital requirements. When you do not eat cholesterol, your body sees this deprivation as a time of 'famine'. During this famine, insulin activates an enzyme in your liver called HMG Co-A Reductase that begins to overproduce cholesterol from the carbohydrates, sugars and insulin producing substances that you eat. The internal production of cholesterol is thought to contribute to the formation of the damaging artery plaque that leads to diseases such as heart attacks and strokes. The only way to switch off the enzyme HMG Co-A Reductase is to eat a sufficient amount of cholesterol daily, found naturally and in nature's bounteous balance, in foods such as eggs, meat, avocado, shellfish and dairy products. (Avoid the foods you many be intolerant to according to your blood type). The body manufactures around 70% of our total cholesterol. Our bodies know exactly how to dispose of unneeded cholesterol when this enzyme is not activated.

So we return to the underlying guiding principles of this programme, which are balance, evolution and natural foods. It makes no sense to me at all that our incredibly developed bodies have not evolved over thousands of years to safely eat what must be one of man's original food sources: eggs, long before he even learnt to hunt. Just a thought. Certainly my clients' bodies and the results support this.

TREATING YOUR HIGH CHOLESTEROL LEVELS... YOU MUST EAT EGGS AGAIN!

If you have high cholesterol, the only way you will balance that level naturally is to start eating sufficient cholesterol to switch the enzyme off, and at the same time significantly reduce your excess sugar and starch intake. This means you can eat as many as 10-14 eggs a week plus some butter and avocado daily, to force the enzyme to shut down! I know, shocking isn't it? After all these years of being told how bad eggs are for you this will seem a complete anathema. But anybody who has stuck to his or her cholesterol-free diet rigidly and still seen their cholesterol levels continue to rise, knows that that approach is flawed. HMG Co-A Reductase is the reason why.

Initially, your cholesterol levels may rise slightly as both the foods and enzyme contribute cholesterol to your body. Your body can manage this, as it will only be for a short space of time. Once the body is reassured that you are eating sufficient dietary cholesterol over a period of around three months, will it switch off the enzyme, and if there are no active viruses in the system, the cholesterol will drop into normal range.

Case History: High Cholesterol
Mike, 60 years old, Blood group O

Mike came to see me in September 2000, because although he enjoyed fairly good health, he did suffer from daily heartburn, low energy levels and a rising cholesterol level that had not responded to a low cholesterol diet. On his doctor's advice, Mike had been strictly avoiding red meat, eggs, butter and cholesterol foods. He led a well-balanced life, played golf regularly, went to the gym twice a week, did not smoke and was careful with his intake of sugar and junk foods. Through his wife's encouragement, Mike had been a vegetarian for five years.

Muscle testing revealed that Mike's food intolerances included wheat, soya, oranges, onions, tomatoes, tea and coffee. Mike immediately eliminated all of these foods, including soya, which had formed a major part of his diet. His heartburn disappeared immediately, but returned as soon as he ate even a small amount of any of the foods I had identified as his intolerances. Within one month, Mike's energy levels had improved substantially and he was feeling much better. To lower his cholesterol, he began to eat two eggs a day, red meat four times a week, butter, avocado and shellfish - all of which his body had requested.

In May 2001, Mike's cholesterol was tested again. To his doctor's surprise, his LDL had dropped significantly and was within the safe zone. His HDL had risen, and his protein and calcium levels were greatly improved. Over the following 2 years, his cholesterol continued to improve, as did Mike's well-being.

I have seen 21 similar cases of patients with high cholesterol, not caused by a virus or toxicity who have been on low fat, low cholesterol diets and who have been taking the statin drug with no positive effect. All of these patients experienced a reduction of their cholesterol levels within four months of beginning this programme.

UNDERSTANDING INSULIN

As we get older, we all develop what is called insulin resistance. Due to our increasingly unhealthy eating and lifestyle habits we are experiencing faster and faster metabolic ageing as our bodies are forced to deal with toxic levels of alcohol, cigarettes, artificial sweeteners, caffeine, poor nutrition, prescription and over-the-counter drugs, chemicals in foods and stress. Because of accelerated metabolic ageing, people are developing insulin resistance at much younger ages than ever before.

Insulin's major function is to regulate bloodsugar levels at all times and protect the brain from receiving too much sugar, which damages the cells. As I have already discussed, insulin is responsible for taking excess sugar out of the blood and storing it in the cells as body fat. Only insulin has this ability. However, our typical diets today are far too high in carbohydrates and we are eating far more than we can use as energy. After many years, influenced also by the health of your cells as a result of other toxic metabolic ageing factors, the cells become saturated with sugar molecules (body fat) and can store no more. They can no longer take in any more sugar. This is known as insulin resistance. Next, the pancreas secretes even more insulin in an attempt to overcome this resistance.

The result is too much insulin in the bloodstream, a condition known as hyperinsulinemia. When the fat cells are filled, the sugar has nowhere to go and remains in the bloodstream. This is Type II diabetes. Type 1 Diabetes occurs when the pancreas stops functioning altogether, usually due to a genetic weakness and commonly occurs in children. This type of diabetes is irreversible.

The Body Talks programme has been highly effective in healing type II diabetes and balancing sugar levels, even in seriously affected diabetics. Because insulin is not triggered to the same extent when you are using protein to slow down the digestion of sugars into the blood, the pancreas gets a chance to rest. As the cells are not being forced to store extra sugar and you are actually taking sugar out of the cells to meet the body's needs, because your dietary intake of sugar is lower, the cells gradually empty. As they empty, the insulin resistance of the cells diminishes and the insulin becomes more effective again. As the pancreas recovers and becomes more efficient, you will notice that your blood sugar level improves without increasing your medication. At this point, and only with your doctor's permission, you may be able to slowly start reducing your dosage. Reaching this stage will take at least three months of careful diet.

Case History: Diabetes
Ahmed, 40 years old, Blood group A

Ahmed was suffering from dizziness, hypoglycaemia (low blood sugar), bad headaches, poor eyesight, numbness in his feet and constant fatigue. He was borderline diabetic, and his body told me that his immune system was working at an average of 51%, and that Diabetes Mellitus II would develop within five months if immediate action was not taken.

Ahmed's body revealed that the main cause of his condition was eating a high carbohydrate diet for many years. I asked him to follow a strict programme, avoiding his food intolerances, and always balancing his protein, low carbohydrate/starch and fat ratio at every meal. I told Ahmed to eat three meals and two snacks a day. His supplement programme included lipase for fat digestion, chromium and biotin.

After six weeks, Ahmed's eyesight had returned to normal and his headaches had gone. His body told me that the diet had enabled his pancreas to heal by 40%. One month later, Ahmed was back to full health and the threat of diabetes had gone altogether. He lost 29lbs/13kg, and looks and feels wonderful.

CHAPTER 4

THE RULES FOR GOOD EATING
THE BODY TALKS

Eating well for life is simply using these following few rules as a daily guideline. Eating a balanced diet over time will naturally heal your weight as your body balances out. Read through this book before you begin your diet so you know the different food types, what they are, and how much of each you should be eating. Then apply these simple rules to every meal you eat.

RULE NUMBER ONE:
EAT PROTEIN LITTLE AND OFTEN AT EVERY MEAL FOR LIFE...

Most of us do not eat enough protein regularly to feed our bodies' needs over the next few hours of the day. During normal everyday activity, a man will use two eggs of protein every 2-3 hours, a woman every 3-4 hours. As the body must have protein every moment, if you do not then eat more, it must break down that precious muscle tissue in order to feed itself. You are then in effect eating yourself from the inside!

As a result, most of us continue to lose muscle mass as we age at a considerable rate.
The average western person is estimated to lose up to 40% of their muscle mass by the age of 60. This means: 40% lower potential metabolic rate; 40% less calories that could be burned up during resting without turning to body fat; 40% less nutrients and goodness to meet your body's daily requirements to stay healthy, which all leads to a downward spiral into ill health.
Eat protein at every meal, breakfast, lunch, dinner and every snack. Do not miss breakfast and ensure you included protein. You will have gone 12 hours without any since dinner the night before. If you miss protein you run the risk of going 17 hours without it.

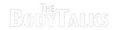

RULE NUMBER TWO
ALWAYS EAT PROTEIN, CARBOHYDRATE AND FATS AT EVERY MEAL AND SNACK

Many of you will be familiar with the 'Food Combining' concept of never eating your proteins and carbohydrates at the same meal. This theory is now 40 years old and was developed by nutritionists when scientists first discovered that proteins were digested by an acidic enzyme and carbohydrates by an alkali enzyme. The theory was that as these enzymes have opposite ph balances, they must cancel each other out. If they did that, then foods would fight when eaten at the same time and not digest properly. Surely this would explain why so many people suffer from bloating and digestive disorders. A sound theory you would think.

Not so. This theory did not take into consideration the effect of fast digestion of sugar and the resulting effect on the liver and sugar levels in the blood. Our bodies have evolved slowly over thousands of years, eating all types of foods at the same time. It made no sense to me that the body would have got this so wrong.

The body explained to me what really happens. We were not put on earth and surrounded by so many good foods to then have nature say: "But if you eat them you will get fat". Mother nature gave us seasons, and certain foods at times of the year when we needed them, another aspect of food that modern life has overcome. She meant us to eat well, to eat plenty and to get all the nutrients we need without starving.

Let us take the example a piece of fruit, an apple, an easy snack that most of us think is healthy, good for weight loss and not fattening. As you now know a medium apple contains approximately three teaspoons of white sugar equivalent in the form of another natural simple sugar called fructose. (One teaspoon of sugar = five grams of carbohydrate). That's a lot of sugar! A banana contains approximately six teaspoons of sugar! (30 grams of carbohydrate).

Now there will be a few trace elements of vitamins and some fibre in the apple, (unless you have just picked the apple off a tree,) but the nutrients and vitamins are already greatly oxidised in most shop

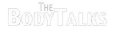

bought fruit, which has travelled across the world. An orange loses as much as 60% of its Vitamin C within 48 hours of being picked. Only traces remain after two to four weeks, which is often how long it takes most of our fruit to reach the supermarket shelves from around the world.

When you eat an apple on its own, it will digest in your stomach very quickly in the absence of any other food. In most fairly efficient stomachs, the fructose sugars in the apple will digest into glycogen and be taken to the liver within 12-15 minutes. **WHAM.** Your liver is suddenly bombarded with 15 grams of sugar. One of your liver's functions is to tightly regulate the amount of sugar reaching the brain at any one time. It rarely needs all that sugar and so is forced to remove some of it from the blood in order to stop your blood sugar level rising too high and reaching the brain, which must remain within a tight sugar range at all times. To do this, insulin will be triggered from the pancreas, whose job is to take sugar out of the blood and store it as body fat. The liver may store some of the extra sugar within itself, as glycogen, if its emergency reserves are low.

The brain is happy as it receives the sugar it needs from the liver. However, there is now insulin present in the bloodstream. It turns from good friend to bad friend, as it then continues to compete with the brain for the available sugar remaining in the blood and as a result drops the sugar level in the blood very quickly. The liver is then forced to compensate by supplying the brain with its store of instant sugar - glycogen - as the level continues to drop. The liver will contain enough glycogen to support the brain and energy needs of the body for around one to three hours, depending on your activity level at the time. Then all the sugar stores begin to run low. The brain, starved of sufficient blood sugar, begins to under-function. You begin to feel very hungry in the pit of your stomach. You may lose concentration, become irritable, feel very sleepy or begin to yawn. Suddenly there is no more available sugar. There is nothing in the stomach, the liver is empty of glycogen, and the extra sugar has already been stored away as very stable body fat.
At this point the brain has two options: it could ideally tell the liver to break down stored body fat to release more glycogen and energy. But the human body has been in famine throughout history, and fat was a very precious commodity which could save your life during long days of starvation. After all,

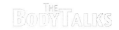

experience has proven time and time again that food can be sporadic during our evolution. You may really need that fat tomorrow. So the first step is to go hunting and see what food is available!

You will start to feel that hunger pang in your solar plexus and begin to crave a food that the body knows will digest rapidly and give it sugar quickly, chocolate perhaps, a croissant, a sandwich, pasta, cake. If it is near lunchtime you will crave that generous portion of starch in the form of pasta or potato or rice or else you think you just won't feel full. It is so important that our brain receives that sugar quickly that the craving is often very powerful and you will be unable to resist it. And the process starts again. The carbohydrates eaten in the absence of, or with insufficient amounts of protein, digest very quickly again. The sugar level soars, insulin kicks in and removes the extra sugar and stores it as body fat or cholesterol. The blood sugar level continues to fall until the next craving hits you around two to three hours later. The craving cycle continues ad infinitum… all day, particularly if you have started your day with a breakfast of 'oh so healthy' fruit, your body's sugar level and brain chemistry yo-yo up and down every few hours.

Your body fat is very slowly but steadily being increased with each meal, your insufficient protein intake results in more and more muscle mass slowly being broken down to meet your metabolic needs and your well being spirals downwards with every new day. Does this ring a bell?

This isn't the only bad news. Dietary fats can ONLY be stored as body fat in the presence of insulin. The insulin released every time you overeat sugar, will also ensure that any dietary fats, happily circulating in the system from the last meal and being put to important use by the many processes needed by the body, are trapped by the insulin and pushed into cells. Like a bossy prison warden, the insulin grabs the dietary fat, converts it to body fat and locks it into your cells.

Innocent fat which would have been normally expelled if not needed through the liver, digestive system and kidneys is now converted into body fat. **FAT DOES NOT MAKE YOU FAT…INSULIN MAKES YOU FAT…** and insulin is triggered in the presence of sugar.

WHAT IS NATURE'S SOLUTION?
TO EAT PROTEIN AT EVERY MEAL IN ORDER TO SLOW DOWN THE DIGESTION OF SUGAR IN THE STOMACH…..

If you eat your apple with some protein and fat, for example, an ounce of cheese, or a couple of slices of ham or cold turkey, the combination of the protein and fat with the sugar in the apple, triggers all the digestive enzymes to be released into the stomach at the same time. Fat triggers bile and lipase, vital enzymes for the proper extraction of nutrients from the other foods.

The protein in the cheese or meat triggers hydrochloric acid, an acidic enzyme, which works against the alkali enzyme glycogen, which responds to the sugar in the apple.

As a result, the apple digests much more slowly over about an hour and the sugar is only released in small amounts to the liver. The liver immediately uses this sugar for the energy requirements of the cells and the brain, your muscles and your daily activity. There is no excess, so nothing is stored as fat or cholesterol. Your body receives an ideal balanced amount of all the nutrients it needs in the form of protein to meet your metabolic need; fat, to act as a catalyst for countless metabolic processes; and sugar for energy. You get to eat twice as many calories and much more food! Your brain chemistry stays balanced and your moods are stable. Your energy levels stay high without any highs and lows. You feel great and you don't put on weight. All in all, your body is perfectly primed for action. Nature is brilliant.

To summarise:
Never eat fruit, sugars, starch or carbohydrate on their own.
ALWAYS combine them.

> **For example…**
> 1 apple and one Babybel cheese
> 1 tangerine and 1oz cold turkey
> 1 banana and ⅓ cup cottage cheese

Or eat one piece of fruit after a meal where you have already eaten protein.

THE BODY TALKS is not a high protein diet. It is a low starch diet. It consists of giving the body exactly the amount it needs to perform at peak output over the hours following a meal. When you eat in the correct ratio of protein, carbohydrate and fat at each meal or snack, every hormone and system in your body is triggered to work at its optimal balanced state. In healthy adults, this ratio is 30-40% protein, 30-40% carbohydrates and 30% fat. Fat occurs naturally in most meats, poultry, dairy foods and eggs in around the 30% ratio. If you are hungry and have low energy two to three hours after a meal, you can be sure you have eaten too much carbohydrate. If you are tired and irritable but not hungry, you will have eaten too much protein. Your body will let you over-eat carbohydrates, but you will not want to eat more protein than you need when you have built up sufficient muscle mass.

In his best selling book 'Enter The Zone', Barry Sears describes how eating in a ratio of actual grams of proteins, carbohydrates and fats of 30:40:30, results in optimal mental and physical performance. By eating in approximately this ratio at every meal, every hormone, biological response and metabolic function works at peak efficiency, leading to freedom from hunger, greater energy and improved mental focus. Many clients bodies have confirmed that this ratio, give or take 5% each way, is the optimal ratio of eating these foods. It does not need to be exact but reminds us to always eat in balance.

Case History: Overweight
Female, age 40, Blood group O+

Having been unable to lose any weight through any type of diet, I first came to see Judy in January 2000 weighing 163lbs and within 3 weeks of following the programme I started to lose weight. I was very strict in following all the advice given and suffered no symptoms of detox; rather I had an abundance of energy and enjoyed exercising. I was delighted when, six months later, I had lost 17lb. I have slipped back a little now as I have not been quite so careful in avoiding my intolerances but am still much healthier and now know how to lose weight healthily and easily if I want to.

RULE NUMBER THREE
EAT PLENTY OF NATURAL FIBRE AT EACH MEAL

Dietary fibre plays a vital role in weight loss and health. High fibre foods slow down the rate at which the stomach empties and therefore the rate at which glucose is absorbed and inhibits the degradation of starch in the small intestine. We all know that a high fibre diet also encourages efficient bowel movements and is scientifically proven to protect the body against degenerative bowel illnesses such as colon cancer and diverticulitus. What is important however is to differentiate good and bad fibre. In prehistoric times, our ancestors foraged on plants which bore little resemblance to today's highly cultivated fruits and vegetables. They rarely ate grains or cereals, which resembled wild grasses rather than the carb-rich cultivated grains we eat today. On average their diets were estimated to contain five times more fibre than our modern diet. With the agricultural revolution, refined white flour became more readily available, stripped of its natural fibre. As wheat became more and more selectively bred and modified, it lost more and more of its natural goodness and became less and less digestible.

Original old fashioned wheat is called Spelt, and most of us who are intolerant to modern wheat, will have no problem with this good old fashioned grain which our ancestors ate for hundreds of years. Other good fibre-rich foods include all the non-starchy vegetables such as lettuce, spinach, cabbage, collard greens, bok choy, alfalfa sprouts, cauliflower, celery, mushrooms, courgettes and herbs such as coriander, parsley, sage, mint, onions, fennel and dill. Where possible, at every meal include a large salad or plenty of vegetables. These will account for most of your carbohydrate needs in the day. Small amounts of whole meal rye or spelt bread or a couple of rye crispbreads also contain excellent natural fibre. These will not only fill you with low-starch nutrient-rich bulk food and improve your bowel efficiency, but will also actively help you lose weight.

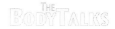

Case History: Constipation
Female, age 45, Blood group A

"Constipation is something you have to learn to live with", so I was told twenty years ago by a Harley Street specialist. Having gone through various undignified examinations and x-rays, the doctor could find nothing seriously wrong except my bowel was now rather stretched, which is not surprising as sometimes I went up to 2 weeks without relief! I grew up being constipated and remember eating all sorts of horrendous mixtures to try and cure me. I was naturally slim but always felt bloated and uncomfortable.

At the time I met Judy I had been eating a high-fibre diet and led a very healthy lifestyle. I had learnt to live with my constipation as I did not want to take laxatives. Judy gave me a list of my food intolerances and I duly omitted these from my diet. Within the first few days I could not believe the change in my system. Everything was working normally and I was no longer bloated. Now, two months later my trousers are getting looser and my legs are slimmer but I have not lost weight on the scales. I know it is still early days but I feel as though all the gunk I have been storing in my body for years is now slowly disappearing! It's not always easy to stick to the diet but my incentive is an amazing increase in energy and well-being, and a flat stomach! It's fantastic to know at last what I can and can't eat.

Aloe Ferox Crystals for Constipation
The most powerful, effective and natural laxative for anyone suffering with chronic constipation is a tiny matchhead amount of the bitter crystal made from the Aloe Ferox Cactus, from the same family as the Aloe Vera plant. Studies in Germany have shown it outperfroms every other natural and allopathic alternative on the market and has no side effects, even when used for many years. I have never sold products unless they are very difficult for my clients to obtain and are amazing enough to warrant a place in my diamond club, available to order on my website at www.judycole.co.uk

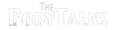

RULE NUMBER FOUR
EAT NATURAL GOOD FATS....

I can't begin to tell you how dangerous low fat diets are for you. Fat is the only substance that registers to our brain when your body has eaten enough. Low fat diets leave you constantly hungry as well as unable to properly process the nutrients from food. Fully skimmed milk should be banned! It is so low in fat, that there is not enough fat in it to trigger the bile into the stomach. Bile, a substance needed to digest fat, is produced in the liver and then stored in the gall bladder. It must be released when milk is drunk to fully digest milk and extract nutrients such as calcium and magnesium. Without it the goodness in milk is passed directly through the digestive system and expelled. Natural fats are vital for proper digestion and absorption of nutrients. Please do not be afraid to eat moderate amounts of natural fats in your diets found in semi skimmed milk, cheese, meats, fish, olive oil, butter (yes butter, see the A-Z for more info), eggs, avocados, nuts and seeds. Eat moderate portions, OFTEN! Your body needs them, which is why they are present in such high amounts in nature!

Case History: IBS

After 5 days on the diet I knew to expect some deterioration in my health as you explained in your sheets. On day 5 my IBS came back with a vengeance, followed a couple of days later with thrush. The IBS has more or less gone away, but the thrush appears to be a little more persistent although not as bad as when it first started. I usually treat myself with Diflucan but wondered if that might not be such a good idea at the moment.

I had a problem with my knees from when I was a child (about 11) up till I was 28 and pregnant the first time. The doctors said it was probably hormonal. Last week I had one really bad day with it and then it disappeared. I also had a problem about 5 years ago with one of my hips, an aching that lasted about 6 months. Last week I had a bad day with that too and then it went away. Cellular detoxing is an amazing experience.
P.A.

RULE NUMBER FIVE
EAT ENOUGH CALORIES….

If you are a woman between 5' and 5'10", you will need an ideal intake of 1600 to 1700 calories a day to lose weight and stay healthy. If you are a man, you will need 1900 to 2000 calories a day. If you drop below this for only around 30 days (according to the body) your starvation mode will kick in, your metabolic rate will drop and your body slows down the utilisation of body fat into energy. On a low fat, low calorie diet, you will initially lose weight on the scales, as you strip your body of muscle mass, bone mass, fluids, brain mass, nutrients and so on. Six weeks later, particularly if combined with an intensive exercise programme, you will become undernourished. Your immune system, controlled by a healthy adrenal gland function, will have fallen even further than when you started your diet; your susceptibility to illness, colds and flu will increase; your moods, controlled by a balance of good nutrients to your brain, will go out of balance.

A lack of vital fats will depress you as your brain becomes starved of fatty acids; you will start to crave sugar. Your body will sabotage your best intentions rather than let you slowly starve yourself and you will rebound and feel the need to eat too much to try and replenish the short fall. You now have a lower metabolic rate than before and a weaker adrenal gland function, which controls your other hormones, fluid retention, immune system, fat metabolism and many other subtle body functions, and absolutely no will power to stop yourself from stuffing food back into your starved body.

Your body goes into overdrive to absorb as many desperately needed proteins, fats and sugars as it can to replace those lost, and your weight piles back on. Have I convinced you never to diet again? On this programme your weight loss graph will look very different.

HOW YOUR WEIGHT LOSS PATTERN SHOULD LOOK....
The following two graphs illustrate how The Body Talks Programme weight loss differs from many low calorie, high carbohydrate, high exercise diets.

The Usual Weight Loss Graph

1. Rapid and significant weight loss due to low calorie eating often combined with an intensive exercise programme.
   Strips body of muscle mass, bone mass, fluids, salts, nutrients and a very small amount of fat.

2. Plateau reached after six to eight weeks, well before ideal weight loss is achieved, usually accompanied by depression, fatigue, perhaps a cold and even flu, due to damaged adrenal glands and immune system and imbalanced brain chemistry caused by insufficient proteins and calories.

3. Body goes into starvation protection mode as metabolic rate drops to a critical point. Demands nutrition urgently and increases appetite, particularly for foods which quickly supply the imbalanced brain chemistry and can be used immediately such as sugar and refined carbohydrates. A lowered metabolic rate ensures maximum retention of minimum calorie intake resulting in accelerated weight gain.

4. Regain of more weight than before due to the further damage done to the immune system, decreased muscle mass, lowered metabolic rate and a further weakened endocrine gland system.

The Body Talks Weight Loss graph

1. Conversion of pound of fat into pound of muscle, no weight loss on scale but noticeable volume loss. You may even see a small gain in weight. Avoidance of food intolerances allows the adrenals to rest and heal, resulting in a stronger immune system, more balanced thyroid and hormonal output and increased vitality. New muscle mass and optimal calorie intake increases metabolic rate.

2. Metabolic rate suddenly leaps about 10% as new muscle mass level is reached, causing sudden drop in weight due to more pounds of fat being burned off than new muscle laid down. Between 3 and 7lbs weight loss may occur in seven to ten days. This is followed by a more gradual weight loss of $\frac{1}{2}$ to 1lb a week as fat loss slightly outpaces the new laying down of further muscle.

3. New critical muscle mass results in a further sudden jump in metabolic rate and Stage Two is repeated. Underlying hormonal imbalances and exhausted adrenals are usually 90% healed by the end of month four. Cases with underlying complications may take much longer.

4. Ideal weight takes time to achieve as deep toxic residues found around the tummy and thighs slowly melt away. If the diet is sustained, you may even go underweight as the body eliminates old cells and tissues. During this time, people report an incredible feeling of well-being and vitality and a reduction in the hours of sleep needed.

5. New tissue and muscle are laid down in a more equal distribution around the body and the typical pear or apple shape becomes more evenly distributed around the body. Cellulite is hugely diminished. The body finally rebalances to its ideal weight with a high muscle mass and low body fat percentage. By now the way of eating on The Body Talks plan has become a way of life and though you may cheat on holidays and at festivities, your body quickly craves a return to the ease and well being of simple, natural good eating habits. This process can take from three to eighteen months.

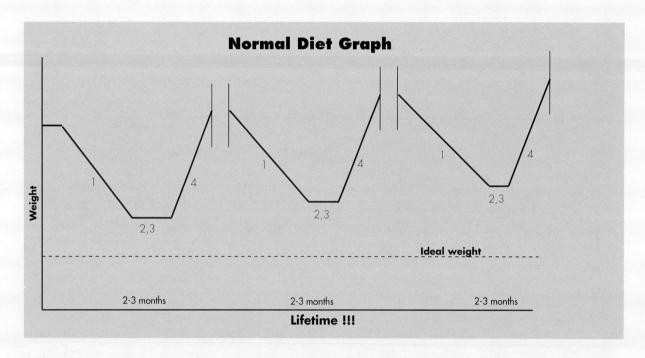
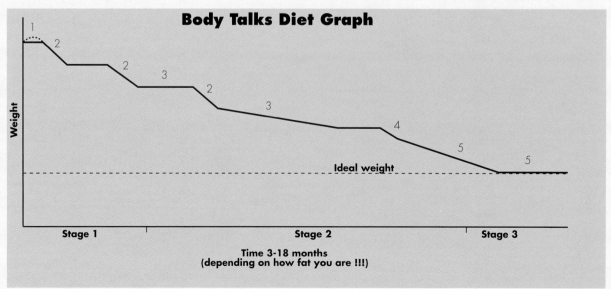

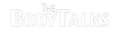

RULE NUMBER SIX
DON'T OVER EXERCISE....

In the early stages of your programme, your priority is to heal your adrenal glands and detox your system. You will need rest and sleep to allow your body the opportunity to do this. During the initial stages of the detox the last thing you will feel like doing is exercising and that's just fine! Toxins also place quite a burden on your system when you exercise. I have never been an excessive exerciser beyond walking my dogs twice a day and swimming two to three kilometres a week. Since detoxing from my food intolerances I noticed a significant improvement in my fitness, without increasing my exercise levels. A year ago I climbed Mount Kinabalu in Borneo with no extra previous training. To my horror I discovered that the climb involved six kilometres of steps on the first day, followed by a midnight steep ascent a few hours later. Several of my companions had trained hard for the event and I was as amazed as they were that I was first to the top. Descending a steep mountain is very strenuous on the legs and I decided it would be far easier to run down as the momentum actually decreases the strain. I set off at a gentle jog with a full back pack and quickly found a rhythm, carefully picking my way down the well maintained rocky steps. For the first time in my life I reached that high that marathon runners talk about and felt I could have gone on and on. It was a feeling that will stay with me for life. I came down in one hour and forty minutes. It took the others nearly four hours to walk it. A few years ago, despite doing much more exercise as a young adult I know I could not have done this. The difference was the lack of toxins in my body. I have consistently noted in the past few years that if I have been eating wheat and try exercising, I am noticeably more sluggish, breathless and red faced. Blood full of excess food intolerance residues is a little like dirty petrol!

Secondly, you are aiming to replace fat with muscle mass. This happens automatically. It is genetically built into your body, a blueprint of muscle shape if you like as long as the body is receiving optimum protein on a regular basis. If you undertake a strenuous exercise routine in these early days, exercising your existing muscles will absorb the very protein that you are hoping to lay down as new muscle. In the first month, it is not advisable to exercise more than a gentle walk, even if you do feel like it. If you are already exercising regularly but have been unable to lose weight, you can be sure you have damaged your endocrine system and will need to dramatically reduce this level to allow your system time and opportunity to heal. If you are not overweight and wish to just undertake the food intolerance detox, reduce your current exercise levels by a third only and resume your previous output after the two months. Too much exercise is well known to be damaging to the immune system. My immune system which I can measure as a percentage function of the adrenal glands by asking my body, sits now after seven years on this programme at a steady 89-91%. (I know, good hey?). The average immune system of people I see ranges from 30% to 60% depending not only on weight and endocrine damage, but the presence of pathogens, toxins and lifestyle.

A few months ago I rode an endurance horse out one morning on a training ride. Unlike my Borneo experience when I felt well and relaxed, I was already stressed and over tired. It was considered an easy day for the horses and we covered around 15 kilometres in about 40 minutes out in the desert, trotting very fast at around 20 kilometres/hour. I had not ridden for some time and though it was thrilling, found it very strenuous. I was exhausted when I got home, and after an hour's sleep dragged myself to work. I was tired for the next two days. On the second day a cold sore appeared on my lip, something I had not had in years since I had been on this diet. I racked my mind for something I had eaten and then finally realised it must have been the shock to my system of the sudden extra exercise to a vulnerable system. It took me two weeks to restore a feeling of well being. Beware of too much exercise if your sensitive glandular system and immune system are compromised and weak when you start this programme.

If you are overweight, sluggish and suffering from any ailments such as headaches, sinus problems, tummy problems and/or low mental state, you can safely assume your immune system is not tiptop! If you do not feel like it or are carrying more than 8kgs of extra weight, you have permission to do NO purposeful exercise for the first month. You will start exercise programme 'A' in your second month on the programme. If you feel fine, are not constantly exhausted and are less than 8kgs overweight when you start this programme, then you may start exercise programme 'A' in the first month.

Moderate activity is sufficient. There will be plenty of time to get fit and tone up later when you are feeling great. Most people, because they feel lethargic and fat, are dragging themselves into gyms and classes in an attempt to use exercise to feel better. Because exercise stimulates the release of the happy hormone, serotonin, we do indeed feel better immediately following exercise, but this is short lived and increasingly addictive. You begin to need more and more exertion to trigger the same serotonin release. In the meantime, inside your body, your tired toxic system is being further damaged. As your immune system drops you become more susceptible to colds and flu, feel increasingly tired between exercise bouts and like John in the story that follows, find that you actually begin to put on weight.

EXERCISE PROGRAMMES

Programme A
Follow for four weeks, building up slowly.

Brisk walking three or four times a week for 20-30 minutes
5 minutes bouncing on the trampoline daily
Optional stretching or yoga/pilates class once or twice a week

Programme B
Follow for four weeks

Brisk walking four times a week for 30-40 minutes
5-10 minutes bouncing on the trampoline four times a week
Optional stretching or yoga/pilates class once or twice a week

Programme C
Follow for Life!

Brisk walking four times a week for 45 minutes
Ten minutes bouncing on the trampoline four times a week
Begin a gentle weight lifting programme over this month but build up very slowly
A stretching or yoga/pilates routine two or three times a week

Follow these three programmes for the first three or four months and then adopt the level of regular exercise that suits you for life. The only strong recommendation I would make is to purchase a small trampoline, a rebounder as they call them, and bounce on it daily for five to fifteen minutes. It increases the blood flow and shunts the blocked lymph around your body, helping with detoxification.

When your immune and endocrine system has reached a point where you feel vital and healthy, free of any ailments, you can begin a more strenuous weight and/or aerobics programme. You may feel that for you, your walking, stretching and bouncing is all you ever need to do for life. For many people this is a sustainable healthy level of exercise that is not too time consuming, requires no special location or equipment other than your bouncer, and can be undertaken into what we now hope will be a healthy old age. If on the other hand you need toning up, would like to shape your body, or just wish to experience a greater level of fitness, your body is now ready to meet this challenge. I would advise you get professional help from a fitness instructor who is not on a mission to turn you into superman or woman in a few weeks, but appreciates the need to build your strength slowly and work with you in always maintaining your health. Changing your body shape requires that you stress the muscle and push the heart, but ensure adequate rest between exercise days and sufficient calories and protein to meet the increased energy needs. Beware that the more body beautiful you aim for, unless you continue to exercise at this level for life, when you do stop, your metabolism goes into free fall and the excess muscle quickly turns back to fat. I would rather maintain a healthy, gentle toned look with a less strenuous regime for life, than pay the price of the backlash in muscle turning quickly back to flab if not maintained at a certain level. (Ask body builders what happens when they stop!).

Don't forget, other wonderful ways of exercising while having fun include cycling, swimming, tennis, squash, rollerblading, hockey, basketball, softball, horse riding, golf, a step class, pilates, indoor wall climbing. Now may be the time to take up a new hobby or reignite the passion for an old one!

You don't ever need to count calories. Ensure you eat 3 good meals and 2 snacks a day of the right foods and the calories will take care of themselves. This programme does not require you to count or measure anything. Eat a healthy balanced diet and enjoy your food.

Case History: Back Ache
Male, age 37, Blood group A

Peter came to see me in January 2001 with constant back pain. Painkillers did not help and scans showed nothing abnormal. After a particularly bad attack Peter had steroid injections which stopped the back pain but then he started getting pain in his arm. His body said that food intolerances were 100% cause of the symptoms.

Two months later I saw Peter again and he was looking great, relaxed and happy. The pain had gone and he was being very careful in following the diet. He had lost two belt holes but his weight had gone up by three pounds, reflecting the deficient muscle mass he needed to replace. He felt and looked younger and much healthier, no doubt also helped by the disappearance of the pain in his back and arm.

Hi Judy,
Hope you are well - thought I would just take this opportunity to thank you for your help and guidance over the past 3 months. Firstly I am pleased to say that my headaches seem to have cleared up and for the first time in years I am living life without painkillers.
I continue to adhere to your eating plan, don't drink tea or coffee at all and try to avoid all wheat products. I feel fitter and healthier than I have in years.

My husband also contacted you last year with two problems. During the past nine months he's managed to give up smoking without putting on a great deal of weight so one problem solved.
Once again many thanks for all your help and advice over the past months.
Best Regards

Anna

Case History: Long term Obesity
John, 32 years old, Blood group A

John first came to seem me in 2000. He was 5'9" and weighed 330lbs (150kgs) and had suffered from obesity since he was 10 years old. His body told me that he was not suffering from a thyroid problem or candida overgrowth, but that his system was sluggish and his adrenal gland was functioning at just 34%. John was 34% protein deficient due to years of eating a high carbohydrate diet and too little protein to sustain his muscle bulk.

Although John had tried every available diet and exercise programme, he had never lost more than a few pounds and had immediately gained weight as soon as he stopped dieting. John quickly understood the simple guidelines of The Body Talks programme, and began a strict detox, eliminating his A blood type food intolerances. John also ate a balanced amount of protein, fat and low-starch carbohydrates, and consumed at least 2000 calories a day. I told John that he must avoid exercise until his exhausted system had been given a chance to rest.

By the time of his follow-up consultation with me a month later, John had lost 9.2lbs (4kgs), but had gone down three belt holes. John could not believe how much he was advised to eat on the programme, nor how his sugar cravings had disappeared. John did feel low in energy, a classic part of detoxing, but felt mentally brighter.

Three months later, John weighed 277lbs (125kgs). His body told me that he had lost 21lbs of actual fat and put on 4 lbs of muscle. His energy was high and his immune system had recovered to a healthier 54%. He was stunned at how easy the programme was and how the weight was falling off him for the first time in his life. At this point he began a light exercise programme, building up to walking for 40 minutes 4 times a week.

Just five months later, John weighed 235lbs (107kgs). He had stuck to the programme rigidly, and had not cheated with his food intolerances more than is allowed. When he returned home to his family that summer, they did not recognise him. He then told me that over the two-month summer vacation, he found he was able to cheat more often and did not regain any weight. His immune and endocrine system had healed so deeply that his body was now able to process excess calories, fat and junk foods occasionally without any adverse effect. John lost a total of 115lbs (52kgs) in 9 months and sustained that weight without any effort, by following the programme.

Then, 18 months after his first consultation, John went to the gym. His personal trainer designed a rigorous weight programme, combined with intensive aerobic exercise three times a week. His body mass index stood at 29%, which is considered overweight, but John was happy with his weight, had no trouble maintaining it and, more importantly, felt fantastic. He was going to the gym to increase his muscle tone and shape. To John's surprise, three weeks into his gym routine his weight began to increase. This was thought to be due to the increased muscle mass he was building, but in fact, his body mass index, his fat to muscle ratio, was also increasing: John was getting fatter again.

When John came to see me recently, almost exactly 2 years after he began my programme, he had regained 15kgs and could not stop it. He had re-damaged his delicate endocrine and immune systems through over-training, and his weight had rebounded. He is now off all exercise other than a 20 minute brisk walk three times a week, and is back on stage one of the programme to re-heal his system.

John lost the weight again and bought himself his dream motor bike, a gift he had promised to himself for years, if he ever reached and sustained his ideal weight.

This case illustrates the fundamental message of this book: you never lose weight through low calorie, high exercise programmes. You can only heal your weight by repairing your endocrine and immune systems.

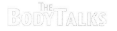

READY, STEADY, GO...

THE THREE STAGES

1. **The first two months-The Cellular detox**
2. **The third month to ideal weight-The Healing Period**
3. **Eating for life-The Maintenance**

> ### Case History: Itchiness, Overweight
> **Brian Age 62, Blood group O**
>
> Brian consulted me in March 2002 with a severe itchy condition over his whole body which he had suffered since childhood. It came on often and suddenly and could last several weeks at a time. The itching would begin on his shoulders and then move down his whole body though there was no visible rash. It was aggravated by cold weather.
>
> His body told me it was a reaction to 60% food intolerances, 10% aftershaves, 10% toothpaste, 10% wool and 10% silk. I use the percentages to make sure I have identified all the culprits and to see what is the biggest cause. The food intolerances included unusual foods such as bananas, onions, bell peppers, sunflower seeds, pistachios, walnuts and caffeine as well as usual O type foods such as wheat, peanuts, tomatoes and spices.
>
> To neutralize the toxic build up and rebalance his overactive but weak immune system the body prescribed itself a powerful supplement programme which included apple pectin which helps bind chemicals in the body and remove them. He embarked on a very strict detox diet.
>
> Two months later he was virtually itch free when I saw him for his follow up he had lost 12kgs of weight, which he had struggled to lose before. He is completely clear of the itching as long as he avoids all of the culprits. Just a short period of time in contact with wool or silk, or a couple of days of cheating on any foods, will set off the itching. As time goes by he seems to be becoming less reactive and is able to tolerate slightly more before getting an attack.

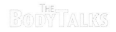

CHAPTER 5

STAGE 1

If you have read the preceding chapters you now have all the necessary knowledge about eating healthily without burdening yourself with in-depth biochemical explanations. If you would like to know more, there is a list of excellent books in the appendix for further reading.

This book is meant to be simple however, and for that reason I am giving you only the information you really need for your new relationship with your body and your eating habits to be effective and easy. My experience has also shown that less is better, in terms of information overload, supplement overload and diet sheets. It is a good idea to keep a diet diary of your progress. This record will prove invaluable to you in the future and help you understand your individual body and needs. To make this easy for you, I have included a ninety day diary in my second book to accompany this programme, called **Vital Food Facts**. This indispensible A-Z answers all the questions I have been repeatedly asked over the years and is vital reading to complete your up-to-date nutritional knowledge. It is a more comprehensive fact-file than the one included in this book.

The cellular Detox

You are now ready to begin your Body Talks Programme. You will have checked your blood type and know which foods you need to avoid for the first two months on this programme. You will have cleared the house of illegal foods and restocked with healthier alternatives that are readily available once you start. You will have informed your nearest and dearest of your intention to get healthy and with any luck they may have opted to join you. You will have weighed yourself and then put away the scales, to get them out **ONLY ONCE A WEEK.** You will understand that, for the first two months, you will need to very strictly avoid your bad foods in order to trigger a cellular detox in your body and clean up your liver and whole system. You will also no longer be frightened of eating lots of good food and good fats, probably more than you have eaten for a long time if you are a seasoned dieter and recognise that regaining your health and shape is a HEALING issue, not one of weight loss. You will need around

1700 calories a day to lose weight slowly but healthily without putting your body in starvation mode if you are a woman, and around 2000 if you are a man. You will not need to weigh or count anything because the basic principles of good balanced eating will take care of that.

For the first two months you will be doing none or only moderate exercise. If you feel well enough and are not more than 10kgs overweight, follow programme one to keep your circulation going and your body supple, and ensure that at no time you stress your immune system. Your body will need the extra energy as it detoxes, to begin to heal itself.

The Rules again…

1. Eat proteins, good carbohydrates and fats at every meal.

2. Eat three meals and two snacks a day.

3. Always eat breakfast. You have gone 10-12 hours overnight without protein.

4. Eat plenty of good fibre each day to fill up on.

5. Eat plenty of good fats in your diet including virgin olive oil, nuts and seeds, fish, avocado and eggs. Do not be frightened of using moderate amounts of butter and never fry anything in any oil, including olive oil or low/fat free spread. Only fry in a little butter.

6. Eat a minimum of 1700 (female) and 2000 (male) calories a day if you are losing weight. Eat 2100 (female) or 2400 (male) to maintain a healthy stable weight.

7. Do not over exercise.

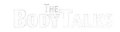

DAILY ALLOWANCES for Stage 1 per day

PROTEINS

Men	**Women**
2 eggs plus two x 6 oz servings of meat, poultry, fish, cheese	2 eggs plus two x 5 oz servings of meat, poultry, fish, cheese

(There is also protein in nuts, pulses and seeds)

COMPLEX CARBOHYDRATES

- Upto 6 ryvita a day-limit to 2 at one meal for women
  limit to 3 at one meal for men
- One slice of rye or spelt bread may be substituted for 2-3 ryvita one meal per day
- One 15g portion of starchy vegetables a day as follows (voluntary)

Each of the following starch vegetable portions contain about 15g of carbohydrate, cooked, the equivalent of three teaspoons of white sugar but very high in fibre and phytonutrients.

Acorn Squash	½ cup	Corn	⅔ cup	Parsnips	⅔ cup
Artichoke	1	Green peas	½ cup	Potato (baked)	medium
Beetroot	1 cup	Leeks	1 cup	Pumpkin	1 cup
Butternut	⅔ cup	Lima beans	½ cup	Sweet potato	½ medium
Carrots	1 cup	Okra	1 cup	Turnip	½ cup

- Two 15g portions of fruit (see page 59)
- One portion of beans or pulses
- Fill up on lots of salads and vegetables, yoghurt
- Use plenty of herbs and mild spices, garlic, ginger and onions to make your meals as appetising as you can

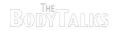

BREAKFASTS: According to your blood type you may eat...

PROTEINS
One of:
- 2 eggs cooked any style
- 1-2 eggs and 2-3 rashers pork or turkey bacon (2-3 times a week only)
- ⅓ cup cottage cheese (not A blood types)
- 2-3oz/50-75g of cold beef (not A blood types)
- 2-3oz/50-75g cold chicken or turkey
- 2-3oz/50-75g smoked salmon, tuna or fish
- 2-3oz/50-75g of feta, halloumi, mozzarella, edam

GOOD CARBOHYDRATES
One of:
- 1-2 Ryvita with butter or Olivio spread
- 1 slice of pure rye or spelt bread
- 1x15g portion of fruit

FATS
Moderate spread of butter or Olive oil spread on bread or Ryvita

DRINKS
- Hot water with the juice of fresh lemon to taste
- Herbal teas such as nettle, camomile, Rooibos, mint, fruit tea
- Dandelion coffee
- Glass of Milk (cow or goat)

Alternative breakfast
BLEND
2 raw eggs, 6oz milk, goats milk or live yoghurt, 1 portion of fruit (½ banana, peach, mango etc) + 1 teaspoon of honey + 1 ice cube.

> 1 cup = 8 fl oz 1 oz = 28 grams

BREAKFAST EXAMPLES:

One of:
- 2 eggs + 1-2 Ryvita or 1 slice rye or spelt bread
- 1-2 eggs + (bacon/turkey bacon) + mushrooms + 2 Ryvita
- 2 egg omelette with cheese/ham + mushrooms/onions/peppers/spinach + 1-2 Ryvitas or 1 portion of fruit
- 2 Ryvita with 2-3oz ham/turkey/beef/chicken/tuna/smoked salmon
- 1 fruit + plain yoghurt + 2 oz cold meat
- 1 fruit + ⅓-½ cup cottage cheese or 2-3 oz feta, mozzarella or halloumi
- 1 smoked mackerel + 1-2 Ryvita or 1 portion fruit

(Always use butter or olive oil spread on ryvita or bread)

LUNCH AND DINNER

Proteins
Women   4-5oz (112-140 grams)
Men   5-6oz (140-168 grams)

These are good guidelines and amount to approximately the size of your palm by one inch thick, or a usual portion of meat or fish. Some days you may want to eat more and others slightly less. This is fine, listen to your body, it will balance out over the week. Your body will never let you eat too much protein, unless you force it.

Any of the following: Smaller portions of one or more can be combined to make up to total recommended protein allowance
- Chicken
- Turkey, duck
- Beef, lamb, pork or veal (not A blood types)
- Salmon, tuna or any fish

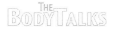

- Prawns, mussels, crab, scallops, lobster, calamari (A and B blood types may eat these only once every two weeks)
- 2-3 eggs (90% of bodies I have asked have said that they can safely eat up to 28 eggs a week with no ill effect, other than becoming sick of the sight of one! You will never want to eat this many but if you are vegetarian then your complete protein options are limited to eggs and cheese and you may choose to eat as many as 4 eggs a day from time to time)
- 2-3oz/50-75g of cheese may be substituted for 2-3oz/50-75g of the above proteins in a mixed salad or where cheese is spread on top of your dish. Pine nuts are also an excellent protein source sprinkled in salads, vegetables and meat dishes.

- **PULSES AND LEGUMES**
  You may include one small portion of beans and lentils once a day if you wish. If you are not losing weight, cut these out and only include them at a later stage. If you are vegetarian, these are vital to balance your daily nutritional needs but must be combined with 1-2 ryvita to make a complete protein.

Carbohydrates:

Unlimited salad with lettuce, (B blood types will prefer Chinese cabbage); rocket, baby spinach, bean sprouts, grated carrot, yellow tomatoes, radishes, herbs such as coriander and mint, a little chopped apple, celery, peeled cucumber (a surprising number of A, O and B blood types are intolerant to cucumber), mustard greens, endive, peppers (also a common intolerance for O and B blood types)

Unlimited cooked vegetables such as asparagus, green beans, broccoli, brussel sprouts, cabbage, cauliflower, courgettes, eggplant (not B blood types), spinach, onions, mushrooms, mange tout.

Vegetables can be steamed, boiled, stir-fried in a little butter, roasted or grilled. Use them in recipes such as stews and mild curries (without tomato).

OPTIONAL STARCH:

One small portion a day of starchy vegetables

and/or 1-2 ryvita with butter or olive oil spread

FATS: 1-2 tablespoons of olive oil as a salad dressing or sprinkled over cooked vegetables

$\frac{1}{2}$ avocado, 3-4 times per week if you like them

Plus: Lemon juice on salads and vegetables

a sprinkling of seeds, nuts or pine nuts.

Remember: *Avoid all potato, sweet potato, rice, corn, wheat free pasta, tortillas, couscous and polenta during Stage 1.*

LUNCH AND DINNER EXAMPLES/IDEAS

- Chicken Caesar salad/Chefs salad with 1-2 Ryvita (optional)
- 2–4 Ryvitas + tuna mayonnaise or egg mayonnaise and/or salad
- Salmon and salad/vegetables
- Steak and salad/vegetables
- 2-3 egg omelette with mushrooms, cheese, spinach, herbs etc
- Roast beef, chicken, lamb, pork with unlimited green vegetables with wheat free gravy. (Use corn flour and gravy browning, avoid Bisto!)
- Stir fries
- Grills
- Stews (thicken sauces with corn or rice flour)

Use plenty of garlic, ginger, herbs, yoghurt, seasoning
Cream is not fattening if eaten with vegetables or protein

HEALTHY CONDIMENTS

    Balsamic and other vinegars
    Garlic
    Low sodium Tamari soy sauce
    Lemon juice
    English and French mustard
    Herbs and mild spices

Remember:

You are learning to listen to your body's needs unless it is craving junk, carbs or sugar. The more you eat of these, the more you will want. Ask your body what it feels like eating every day and try and bring balance and variety into your diet where possible.

Please note:

Avoid all diet and low sugar foods which will contain aspartame or saccharine, the chemical sugar substitutes. They are very poisonous and actually cause weight gain and bloating as they encourage the body to withhold excess water. See Food Tips on page 134 for further information on these substances.

Avoid smoked and processed meats.
Avoid all processed refined margarines and oils; use **ONLY** butter, olive oil spreads and virgin olive oil.

SNACKS

Snacks are vital as they convince the body there is plenty of food around and it can switch off the famine mode. Snacks balance your brain chemistry and stop sugar cravings and they make a vital contribution to your calorie intake requirements for the day.

It is very important to eat every three to four hours. You need to feed your body often in order to win back its trust and reassure it that you are no longer living in a famine. Even if you are not hungry, eat a little something to reassure your body that food is available. This triggers it to turn off the famine mode and increase the metabolic rate. If you are eating breakfast before 8.30 in the morning and will not be eating lunch before 1.00pm, eat a snack mid morning around 11.00am. If you are at work and find stopping for a break impossible, keep a bag of almonds in your desk or car and grab a small handful of only 6-10 nuts. Snacks will also ensure that your blood sugar level stays even and that you are not starving or craving a quick carbohydrate fix by the time you go to lunch. The gap between lunch and dinner for most people is around 7 to 8 hours, far too long for any self-respecting body!! By the time you eat dinner your sugar levels are low, you are tired and irritable and you are likely to feel the need for starches to fill you up. This is a message from the brain demanding quick sugars to top up the plummeting blood sugar levels. By eating a good sized snack around 4-5 pm, you ensure the blood sugar level stays balanced and sugar cravings do not set in. Snacks are also vital to keep your calorie intake up. See the suggestions below for quick easy balanced snacks. In emergency, another small handful of almonds is better than nothing.

TIPS
Fridge at home: Tuna or egg mayonnaise, roast meat, chicken or turkey that can be put on rye crispbread for a quick snack.

Office: Almonds, plain yoghurt and honey, mozzarella cheese sticks, fruit, rye crispbread, cold meat, chicken or turkey.

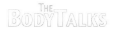

SNACKS EXAMPLES: ONE OR MORE OF THE FOLLOWING AT ANY SNACK
(You could have one of each if you are hungry!)

- 6-8 almonds
- Plain live yoghurt + 1 teaspoon honey
- 1-2 Ryvita + cold meat/tuna/egg/hummus/smoked salmon
- 1 fruit + 2 oz cold meat or $\frac{1}{3}$ cup cottage cheese or 2 oz cheese
- Vegetable crudités such as celery, peppers, peeled cucumber + $\frac{1}{3}$ cup of hummus

LIQUIDS AND DRINKS

- ✓ Try and drink little and often, approximately 1½ to 2 litres of water a day. Add a little lemon juice to taste as often as possible.
- ✓ Water down fruit juices. Add $\frac{1}{3}$ juice to $\frac{2}{3}$ water, soda or fizzy water. Do not drink too many carbonated drinks as these can affect the sodium/potassium balance in your body and cause bloating.
- ✓ Unlimited herbal teas
- ✓ Dandelion coffee

(Only the A blood-type can tolerate coffee and black teas, but even they should limit themselves to no more than 3 cups of either per day)

Liquid Measures (approximate equivalents)

Metric	Imperial	Metric	Imperial
62ml	2 fl oz	250ml	½ pint
125ml	4 fl oz	375ml	¾ pint
125ml	¼ pint	500ml	1 pint

DAILY FRUIT INTAKE

The body recommends no more than two portions of fruit a day. To remind you of the amount of sugar in different fruits, here is the table again for quick and easy reference.

All fruits are raw, except where noted. Each of the following natural carbohydrate portions contains 15 grams of carbohydrate.

Apple	1 small	*Lychees	7 fruit
Apples (dried)	3 rings	*Mangoes	½ medium
Apricots	2 medium	Melons (cantaloupe)	1 cup (cubes)
Apricots (dried)	7 halves	Melons (honeydew)	1 cup
Avocado (large)	½ fruit	Nectarines	1 medium
*Bananas	½ medium	*Papayas	½ cup (mashed)
Blackberries	¾ cup	*Passion fruit	3 fruits
Blueberries	¾ cup	Peaches	1 medium
Cherries	8 cherries	Pears	½ large
Cranberries	1 cup	Pears (dried)	1 half
Currants (dried)	2 tablespoons	Pineapple	2 slices
*Dates	2 medium	Plums	2 fruits
*Figs	2 medium	*Pomegranates	½ fruit
*Figs (dried)	1 medium	Prunes	2 prunes
Grapefruit	½ large	Pomelo	¾ cup
•Grapes (large)	7 grapes	Raisins (seedless)	2 tablespoons
•Grapes (small)	10 grapes	Raspberries	1 cup
*Guavas	1½ fruit	Rhubarb	7 stalks
*Kiwi fruit	1 large	Strawberries	1½ cup
Lemons	3 medium	*Watermelon	1½ cup (dice)
Limes	2 medium		

* denotes should be avoided by A blood types
• Should be avoided if detoxing from yeast

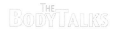

ALCOHOL

A tough one but if you can abstain from all alcohol for the first two months the pay off is huge! If you are drinking alcohol the whole detoxification process is slowed down due to the burden on the liver. Alcohol is full of calories and super sugars which trigger huge amounts of insulin. The human body was not designed to drink alcohol regularly. Alcohol accelerates metabolic ageing, kills off brain cells, causes high cholesterol, blocked arteries, cellulite, diabetes, brain chemistry imbalances, bloating, sugar cravings, mood swings even when not drinking, thyroid imbalances, female hormone imbalances and of course weight gain. But then you knew that didn't you!

If you are drinking every day, even a single glass of wine, your liver never gets a long enough break to detox and the long-term effect of the drip drip of alcohol constantly into your liver is very damaging to your health. If you are a regular drinker try and adopt a policy of not drinking for four consecutive days a week, to give your body chance to fully detox. Ideally, limit your alcohol intake to no more than four to five units a week in the long term. All alcohol contains yeast for fermentation.

Alcoholic drinks:

	Measure	Calories	Carbohydrate (gms)
Beer	½ pint	148	13.2
Sweet white wine	3.5oz	153	11.4
Sweet Cider	7.0oz	136	29.0
Dry white wine	3.5oz	80	3.4
Red wine	3.5oz	76	2.5
Champagne	3.5oz	70	2.2
Malt whiskey	1 shot	70	–
Vodka	1 shot	70	–
Rum	1 shot	70	–
Other Spirits	1 shot	70	–

Best of a bad bunch

Alcohol	Calories
Tequila and lime	70
Campari and Soda	70
Dry white wine and soda	80
Champagne	70

BEWARE: Although the alcohol may not be high in sugar, it has a very high glycaemic index, meaning it enters the blood stream very quickly and over stimulates insulin production, which means the calories quickly turn to body fat. The calories and sugars are also very high in the mixers…

Mixer	Measure	Calories	Carbohydrate(gms)
Coke	8oz	108	27.0
Fruit-flavoured sodas	8oz	119	30.5
Apple juice	8oz	116	29.0
Orange juice	8oz	111	26.0

FOR EXAMPLE…

Vodka and orange		181 calories
Rum and coke		178 calories
Pint of lager	16oz	197 calories

STAGE ONE
FOOD FOR THE DAY

Breakfast:

Either
- 2 eggs (any style) + 1-2 Ryvita **or** 1 slice rye or spelt bread (with butter/olive oil spread)

or
- 1-2 eggs + bacon/turkey bacon + mushrooms + 1-2 Ryvita **or** 1x15g portion fruit
- 2 egg omelette + cheese/ham/mushrooms/onions/peppers/spinach/chives/coriander + 1-2 ryvita
- 2 Ryvita with 2oz ham/turkey/beef/chicken/tuna/smoked salmon
- 1 x 15g portion fruit + plain yoghurt + 2 oz cold meat
- 1 x 15g portion fruit + 1/3-1/2 cup cottage cheese
- 1 smoked mackerel + 1-2 Ryvita or 1x 15g portion fruit
- 2 raw eggs, 6oz milk or live yoghurt, 1 portion of fruit (1/2 banana, peach, mango etc) + 1 teaspoon of honey + 1 ice cube.

Snacks:
One or more of:
- 6-8 almonds
- 2-3 oz plain live yoghurt + 1 teaspoon honey
- Ryvita + 2oz cold meat/tuna/egg/hummus/smoked salmon
- 1 x 15g portion of fruit + 2oz cold meat or 1/3 cup cottage cheese or 1-2oz cheese
- Veggie sticks + hummus

Lunch and Dinner:

Protein | Women 4-5oz/110-140g
| Men 5-6oz/140-170g

e.g. | average size serving of poultry, fish, meat or 3 eggs
or | mix and match e.g. 2oz cheese + 2-4 oz meat/fish/chicken

Plus | Unlimited vegetables grown above the ground and/or salad
Optional | One 15g portions of root vegetables a day
(avoid starches while on weight loss including potato, rice and corn)
One portion of pulses, beans or legumes
1-2 ryvita at each meal (maximum 6 pieces per day)

Use plenty of olive oil and lemon/vinegar dressing, garlic, herbs and seasoning in your food to make it interesting. A little cream can be used on vegetables and meats.
Include $1/3$-$1/2$ avocado 3-4 times a week if you like them

Nuts and seeds already contain a balance of protein and carbohydrate and a small serving can be included in any meal without altering the balance of the rest of your meal

CHAPTER 6

STAGE TWO
MONTH THREE TO IDEAL WEIGHT

THE HEALING STAGE

After the first two months, you should begin to feel like a new person. Many people look so different after the two months that friends think they have had a face lift! You will have lost some fluid and that bloated feeling and your energy levels will be on the rise. You will have lost volume but may not have lost as many pounds on the scales as you want because as quickly as you have lost a pound of fat, you have replaced it with a pound of firm healthy muscle tissue. Your volume will have changed, however, and you will be feeling and looking much better. Still a way to go though if you were very overweight to begin with. Permanent weight loss takes time in order to HEAL the damage. I have noticed that many conditions, whether weight loss or healing a digestive, skin or any disorder that has been with you for a long time, can take as long as nine months to heal deeply, though significant improvements are usually seen within three months. A rebirth almost! You must be patient and make this a way of life. If you abuse in excess ever again, you will gain weight again. There is no magic pill against bad habits and weight gain, as they will just re-damage your system.

In the next stage, you may reintroduce a very small amount of good starch carbohydrates such as brown rice, jacket potato, corn on the cob, whole grains such as millet or oats and up to two slices of whole rye or spelt bread, once a day. Some people find that this slows down their weight loss again whereas others notice no difference. However, if you have a lot of weight to lose you may opt to stay on the first stage until you have lost a little more. It is important however, that no matter how overweight you are, you reintroduce some starch and sugars within three months as our bodies need a little and without it, you may start to crave them in excess again.
However, it must be a balance, or the more you have, the more you want.

If at any time you start to crave them again, you must stop them all, look closely at your protein intake, and ensure you are eating in balance. If you are very strong willed, two little pieces of dark chocolate, preferably around 70% cocoa solids, may be eaten a few times a week from stage two onwards. Be careful, although this little will do no harm, do not let it become a slippery slope. Often this is enough just to satisfy that sweet craving before it becomes a binge but must always be eaten after a meal, never on its own.

In the third and fourth month your body will begin to heal very deeply. Your adrenal glands, relieved of the burden of food intolerances, are able to rest and recover. Your body's ability to metabolise fats, rid itself of excess fluids, balance your hormones and utilise energy in the cells will improve. Your general well-being will continue to increase and your body shape will continue to change. If you find your shape and weight have reached a plateau for more than four weeks, you can shock your system by reducing your food intake for one week only. By cutting the calories down to 1200 calories for no more than 8 days, your weight will begin to drop again. However, if you stay on too low an intake of calories for any longer than this, you risk switching on the famine mode again and your body will hang on to all its extra weight. Do not repeat this low calorie week more than one week in every four. To cut your calories, reduce your portions of everything but you must continue to eat three meals plus two small snacks a day. Avoid nuts during this 1200 calorie week as they are high in calories. Ensure you take an Alfalfa supplement during this week. See page 129.

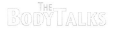

Additions to Stage One

You may add just one of the following meal options at **either** breakfast, lunch or dinner to the stage one menu daily, until you have nearly reached your target size or weight. At that time you can then move onto the stage three programme which is maintenance for life.

ONE OF...

Alternative breakfast options:
- ⅓ cup of oatmeal + milk/water with butter and cream with only 1 teaspoon honey + 2oz cold meat or 2 eggs
- A small bowl of wheat free cereal with milk + 2oz cold meat or 2 eggs

Or in addition at lunch or dinner
- 1 small potato or sweet potato (about the size of a tennis ball)
- 2 tablespoons brown rice
- 2 tablespoons wild rice
- 1 tablespoon white rice (bad option)
- 2 tablespoons of wheat free pasta such as corn, rice or millet
- 1 tablespoon sweet corn
- 2 corn tortilla
- 1 slice whole rye or spelt bread
- 1-2 ryvita

Your carbohydrate intake must always be eaten with protein, fats and unlimited vegetables and salad.
i.e. Never eat fruit on its own, always combine it with some protein.
Pulses, beans, nuts and seeds already contain a mix of protein and carbohydrate and can be added to any meal without altering the balance of the rest of your meal.

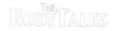

Case History: Severe Dermatitis
Kate Kernick, Blood group O

In the couple of months since I first saw Judy I am finally rid of chronic eczema on my hands. For four years I had tried everything I could think of to bring it under control, and being a holistic nutritionist I ultimately became despondent when I realized I couldn't heal myself. As Judy revealed, I was completely on the wrong track. When she did my reading my body told her I had a severe contact allergy to stainless steel. Not only was it affecting my hands but it was seriously damaging my immune system; it was running at 40%. Also, some of the foods I was eating were weakening my stomach and my lumbar region in my back. There weren't all that many but they were wreaking havoc: wheat, dairy, tomatoes, oranges and tropical fruit which follows consistently with foods to avoid for type A blood types. I changed my diet immediately, avoided stainless steel like the plague and although I fell off the wagon every now and then I was absolutely determined to regain my health. During my initial couple of months detox I did the liver cleanse. All up I counted around 200 stones (some rocks, some pebbles!) and I could hardly believe my eyes at what had been stuck in my liver. For our bodies' sake I really recommend doing this cleanse and you will be astounded by the results.

Initially my body told Judy I would need 9 months to completely clear my system of stainless steel build up, boost my immune system and return to full health. However, just 2 months later when I saw her again my left hand had completely healed after years of peeling and my right hand had just a few small dry patches on it. My body only needed another couple of weeks before my skin was completely healed and my immune system was already running at 73% up from 40%. My stomach was almost 100% healed. The human body has the most incredible ability to heal itself, given the chance. With eternal thanks to Judy, and after all this time I am so thrilled that my hands look so normal again and I don't feel ashamed of them. My quest is not quite over though; I am still researching what it is about stainless steel in particular that makes my body react to it in such a damaging way.

(I have three other clients with severe reaction to stainless steel. One gets very bad itching all over, the other terrible headaches and most surprisingly the third has suffered with uncontrollable blood pressure at the age of only 36. She only has to hold a knife and fork for 60 seconds for her BP to go through the roof. She now uses silver cutlery and her BP has finally stabilized! Judy).

STAGE TWO
FOOD FOR THE DAY

Breakfast:

One of:
- 2 eggs (any style) + 1-2 Ryvita **or** 1 slice rye or spelt bread (with butter/olive oil spread)
- 1-2 eggs + bacon/turkey bacon + mushrooms + 1-2 Ryvita **or** 1x15g portion fruit
- 2 egg omelette + cheese/ham/mushrooms/onions/peppers/spinach/chives/coriander + 1-2 ryvita
- 2 Ryvita with 2oz ham/turkey/beef/chicken/tuna/smoked salmon
- 1 x 15g portion fruit + plain yoghurt + 2 oz cold meat
- 1 x 15g portion fruit + $1/3$-$1/2$ cup cottage cheese
- 1 smoked mackerel + 1-2 Ryvita or 1x 15g portion fruit
- 2 raw eggs, 6oz milk or live yoghurt, 1 portion of fruit ($1/2$ banana, peach, mango etc) + 1 teaspoon of honey + 1 ice cube.

Extra options
- $2/3$ cup of oatmeal + milk/water with butter and cream + 2oz cold meat or 2 eggs
- Small bowl of wheat free cereal with milk + 2oz cold meat or 2 eggs

Snacks:
One or more of:
- 6-8 almonds
- 2-3 oz plain live yoghurt + 1 teaspoon honey
- Ryvita + 2oz cold meat/tuna/egg/hummus/smoked salmon
- 1 x 15g portion of fruit + 2oz cold meat or $\frac{1}{3}$ cup cottage cheese or 1-2oz cheese
- Veggie sticks + hummus

Lunch and Dinner:
As stage one

Extra starch allowance at either lunch or dinner

One of:
- 1 small potato or sweet potato (about the size of a tangerine)
- 2 tablespoons of brown rice (cooked)
- 2 tablespoons of wild rice
- 1 tablespoon of white rice
- 2 tablespoons of wheat free pasta such as corn, rice or millet
- 1 tablespoon of sweet corn
- 2 small corn tortilla
- 1 slice whole rye or spelt bread
- 1-2 ryvita

- Use plenty of olive oil and lemon/vinegar dressing
- Include $\frac{1}{3}$-$\frac{1}{2}$ avocado 3-4 times a week

If you include your starch allowance, do not also have ryvita

CHAPTER 7

STAGE THREE
EATING FOR LIFE

Well done! You have reached your ideal weight. Remember that your ideal weight may still be heavier than you would like, but it is a weight at which you look and feel healthy. It is a weight that you should be able to sustain without too much effort, and that makes you feel good about yourself. It is a waste of energy and self esteem to try and reach the weight you were when you were twenty one, ten years later. Our bodies change naturally as we get older. Be realistic and be happy.

Now, how do you maintain your weight for life?

Firstly, avoiding a long term build up of your food intolerances again is the fundamental secret to supporting your immune system. Try not to eat them more than once every three to four days, to allow any residue to clear from the blood and cells rather than build up a residue. You will find that some of your food intolerances will affect your well being within a short time of eating them resulting, hopefully, in a natural tendency to avoid them. Others will have no effect if you eat a little but the slippery slope begins and before you know it you are eating them daily. Modern day wheat is the worst offender. You will feel fine for a few weeks or even months and then slowly realise that your well being and vitality has dropped again or that some of your old ailments are returning. Most people, including myself, fall off the wagon about three times, before it slowly dawns on us that it is far less painful to permanently adopt alternatives than to suffer the consequences.

Reaching a weight you are happy with may have taken you as long as nine months to a year if you had a lot of weight to lose. Even if it has only taken you three or four months, you will now be very familiar with the basic ways of eating well for life. This is not a diet programme remember, this is a way of eating for life that our ancestors and grandparents followed. You have just returned to good habits and good natural foods. We have been so brainwashed by food manufacturers and advertising into buying processed foods that we believe that our way of eating these days is healthy and that somehow by eating simple, natural foods, we are depriving ourselves. Boy, have those marketing guys done a good job! The secret of long term health and weight control now is to adopt this way of eating as a general rule but allow yourself the occasional day off with a yummy dessert, weekly food intolerance and even binge on special occasions.

We are after balance. Once you have reached your ideal weight, you will need an extra two to four hundred calories a day to stop yourself losing too much. This will be obtained from increasing the number of small starch portions you eat a day. Or you can add a little soul food. A little ice cream or dessert a few times a week is not going to do any harm. Over-indulge regularly and you will put the weight back on!

Most of us do not eat out in expensive restaurants very often. If you are unlucky enough to find yourself eating out regularly for business or for whatever reason and being tempted by rich indulgent menus often, ignore the following advice and be as strict as you can. For those of us for whom a lovely restaurant is more of a treat, my general rule is to enjoy it when you are there. Because I am aware of how awful I could feel the next day if I go overboard, I will stay within my intolerances where possible on the main course and cheat on the starter or dessert. I find I can rarely eat all three courses and as I have a sweet tooth prefer the dessert, but often I will have a starter only to find to my horror that I have no room for a dessert! If you do eat out regularly, you are going to have to watch yourself and be very strict most of the time. The next chapter covers your options for eating out at six different cuisines, to help guide you. Too many dinners or too many courses of rich food, even if you are avoiding your intolerances, will catch up with you.

Studies have shown that people who stay in the region of their ideal weight for life do not have a magic metabolism or body type. They manage their weight better. They watch their weight like hawks and if they put on only one or two pounds, immediately cut down again until they get rid of them. People with a tendency to be overweight, particularly if they have fought a weight problem all their lives, allow the pounds to creep on and only begin to take action when they look fat and have become significantly overweight. If you have been one of the latter to date, get your scales out now that you have achieved an acceptable body, and monitor yourself daily. Set yourself a limit of two pounds over the weight at which you now find yourself happy to stay at. If your weight creeps up, take immediate action and re-

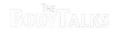

adopt the Stage 1 programme until you have lost it. No buts! As your body becomes healthier and less toxic during the first two stages of the programme, you will find it easier to 'read' your body's nutritional and calorie needs. No longer controlled by brain imbalance and cravings, your body increasingly enjoys the fresh light taste of natural, healthy foods. This reaction becomes instinctive and you will find that you know if those pounds have crept on without getting on the scales.

It is the festive seasons or summer holidays that are generally our undoing. Due to the pressures to keep eating too many wrong foods over these periods, we over-ride our body's early warning signs and stuff ourselves anyway. Within no time, the carbohydrate addiction kicks in, our brains become less balanced and getting disciplined again is a huge effort. If you do lose it, set a date to get back onto Stage One as soon as you can after such a binge and stick to it.

From now on you may have one of the starch options from Stage 2 at **each** meal during the day, but become aware of your particular metabolic rate and body type. For some people, even this amount of starch may cause them to put weight back on and you would need to limit yourself to having starch at just two meals a day. For others, particularly if you are exercising regularly and actively, you may even need to increase the portions at each meal. In stage 3 it is important you remain flexible and adjust your intake according to your current lifestyle. Now you understand how food works, use that knowledge to eat according to your body type. To remain at your ideal weight, the secret of eating starch is to limit the portions even if you eat a little three times a day. Keep in mind that one tablespoon of white rice is three teaspoons of sugar; a plate of pasta, even wheat free, will contain as much as twenty teaspoons! If you are out for dinner, either have starch in the form of rice or potato, OR have a dessert. If you are having a glass or two of wine, remember this is also sugar.

OPTIONAL EXTRAS TO FEED THE SOUL

In Stage 3, you may now add a portion of any **ONE** of the following, eaten **ONCE DAILY** to the programme, **4-5 times a week,** without any bad effects. This will complete the weight maintenance programme for life. Remember these are sugars and must always be eaten with some protein or after a meal. If you eat these too often your weight will creep up again, unless your exercise is increased to counteract it.

Either	Flapjack (Oat and honey bar)
or	Small bar or upto 6 pieces of chocolate eg. small Mars Bar size
or	Moderate portion of wheat free dessert or ice-cream
or	Small piece of wheat free chocolate cake (See appendix for recipe)
or	One bag of potato hoops or crisps (chips)

OTHER INTOLERANT FREE OPTIONS

Wheat free desserts:

Chocolate mousse
Meringues
Cheesecake without the biscuit base
Ice cream
Frozen yoghurt
Sorbet
Fruit and plain yoghurt

Lactose Free desserts

Dark chocolate mousse
Meringue and fruit
High quality Ice cream made with real cream (e.g., Haagen Das, Baskin Robbins, Ben and Jerry's)
Frozen yoghurt
Sorbet

Remember: Always eat these foods with protein to slow down the digestion of the sugar.

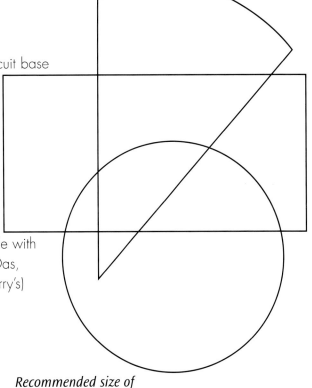

Recommended size of dessert portion

EATING OUT

This need not be the problem you might imagine if you choose your restaurants carefully or know what to ask the chef to prepare for you if there really is nothing on the menu. The biggest difficulties in sticking to the programme occur when you are caught out during the day and need to eat quickly.

The following are good options to look for on menus or to ask the chef to prepare specially for you. These are simple dishes and most restaurants are happy to try and oblige. Many chefs will thicken freshly made sauces with corn flour instead of wheat. Ask if they can do you a small portion of brown rice instead of white rice. The more of us who ask for what we need, the more awareness will increase for the need for these healthy options on menus. Don't be afraid to ask!

Do not allow yourself to be tempted by bread baskets. Request that they be taken away or preferably never delivered. Hot restaurant bread is a wicked temptation and I defy anyone to sit there and resist it when it is sitting in front of you. But resist it you must, especially in the first two months of your programme.

Other good tips
Do not arrive at a restaurant starving. Before you go out, snack on some almonds, a hard boiled egg or a few slices of cheese with half an apple to take the edge off your appetite. If you are being careful with your snacks you should not ever reach a point of being very hungry anyway. A couple of glasses of water will also help fill you up.

- Request extra vegetables or salad instead of rice, potato, pasta or bread.
- Be as strict as you can but don't torture yourself if you accidentally or unavoidably have to cheat. It is only one meal and you will detox within a day. If you are in the first two months of your detox, cheating will stop your body detoxing for five days but will not be enough to rebuild any toxic residue: regular cheating will.

Here are some good options to look for on menus

Starters
- Soups, even if thickened with a little wheat flour and eaten only occasionally, will not contain enough of it to do you any harm
- Warm goat's cheese salad
- Arabic mezze but avoid the deep fried kofta and pastries. Hummus, tabouleh, moutabel with salads are excellent
- Grilled vegetables with cheese or parmesan
- Smoked salmon or cold meats with side salad
- Asparagus
- Prawn cocktail with dressing on the side. Add just a teaspoon or two for flavour rather than drowning it

Main Courses
- Grilled fish, salmon, chicken, lamb chops, steak with a large side salad and/or vegetables
- Roasts, carvery (No Yorkshire puddings! During stage 1, avoid roast potatoes and fill up on meat and vegetables. The gravy will be thickened with wheat flour so only have a little)
- Stir fries, (ask them to substitute rice or rice noodles instead of pasta and then ensure you only eat a maximum of two tablespoons of these. If you are in your strict weight loss phase, do not have any)

CUISINES FROM AROUND THE WORLD

Here are some good suggestions and things to avoid in six different cuisines. Try and only have two courses, either a starter if you are dieting or a dessert if you are on maintenance, with your main. Within these choices choose according to your blood type and ask if you are not sure about the ingredients.

Arabic Restaurants

Choose
- Hummus and vegetables
- Moutabel
- Grilled shish lamb or chicken kebabs
- Kofta (balls of ground lamb and onions, skewered and grilled)
- Mint tea

Avoid
- Pitta bread
- Tabouleh (contains wheat and tomatoes)
- Fattoush
- Kibbe
- Falafel

Chinese Restaurant

Choose
- Egg drop soup
- Barbequed spare ribs
- Fish, prawns, chicken or beef with mushrooms and bamboo shoots.
  With walnuts or cashews
  With lemon sauce
  With vegetables
  With garlic sauce
- Mixed vegetables
- Plain boiled rice (if not on strict diet)

Avoid
- Spring rolls
- Dumplings
- Crispy egg rolls
- Crispy duck in pancakes
- Sweet corn soup
- Oyster, sweet and sour, black bean, honey and soya sauces
- Chow mein
- Noodles
- Fried rice

French restaurants

Choose
- Coquilles St Jacques (scallops in cream sauce with cheese)
- Frisee salad with lardons (thin strips of bacon-optional) and poached egg
- Moules mariniere (mussels in white wine)
- Bouillabaisse (fish stew)
- Smoked salmon and asparagus
- Steak au poivre, tournados Rossini (beef stuffed with pate and mushrooms), steak chasseur (contains small amount of tomato), Bourdelaise sauce (reduced shallot and red wine sauce)
- Coq au vin
- Vegetables in butter or cream
- Mousse au chocolat (if not on strict weight loss programme)
- Pavlova (if not on strict weight loss programme)

Avoid
- Tomato based sauces
- Pastry
- Vichyssoise (cream of potato soup)
- Potato dishes such as Duchesse, Gratin Dauphinois or Savoyarde (all excess carbohydrate cooked with cream, cheese or butter)
- Croque monsieur (bread dipped in egg and fried with ham and egg)
- Quiche (Unless you remove the pastry)
- Crepes

INDIAN RESTAURANTS

Choose
- Mild tandoori marinated chicken or prawns
  i.e. Any meat in a mild marinade made from yoghurt or cream
- Tandoori gobhi (cauliflower marinated in tandoori masala)
- Dal
- Paneer shish kabab (cottage cheese seasoned with herbs and barbequed on skewer.)
- Paneer garlic tikka (any paneer which is not fried)
- Mutton keema (minced mutton cooked with spices)
- Mutton or chicken bhuna (cooked dry with spices)
- Mutton or chicken mughlai (dry cooked and garnished with egg)
- Dahi (plain yoghurt)
- Maximum two tablespoons boiled rice (if not on strict diet)

Avoid
- All curry sauces are tomato based and must be avoided strictly for the first three months on your detox. When made at home, tomatoes can be substituted with tamarinds. After that, you can eat them once every four to five days in a curry, if you are not also having them in salads.
- Pakora
- Samosa
- Poppadom
- Curry sauces
- Naan
- Paratha
- Roti

Italian Restaurants

Choose
- Beef carpaccio
- Caesar salad
- Seafood salad
- Melon and parma ham
- Cream of vegetable soups such as courgette, mussels, country vegetable
- Mozarella with basil and balsamic dressing (without tomatoes)
- Grilled chicken paillard (boneless chicken, pounded thin), piccata or scallopini.
- Fresh fruit
- Ice cream (not if on strict diet)
- Cheese board - substitute biscuits with a piece of fruit

Avoid
- Deep fried calamari
- Deep fried camembert
- All pasta
- Risotto (if on weight loss programme)
- Lasagne
- Pizza
- Tiramisu

Mexican Restaurants

Difficult!! I looked at their menus and everything has something illegal in it, except the fajitas, the plain sizzling meats which you can eat with salad, refried beans, avocado and cheese. When you have achieved your goal on this programme then treat yourself to a blast, but beware, you will feel terrible afterwards! By the way… Tequila is the only alcohol without any yeast in it and if you like it, is usually the only alcohol that won't give yeast intolerees a hard time! Still just as calorie laden though.

Fast Food

There are times in our busy lives where fast food is your only option. Try and avoid it by being prepared and keeping a bag of almonds with you at all times in case of hunger emergency. Do not cheat on fast foods in the first three months of the programme, think ahead and take food with you, including on aeroplanes.

You will, I hope, be well aware of the huge amount of saturated fat, calories, salt, sugar and lack of nutrition in most fast foods. What you may not be aware of is:

- Most fast foods are fried in oils which have been reheated many times. They are rancid and highly toxic.
- Many fast foods are made from substandard foodstuffs, such as offal and bone scrapings in beef and chicken burgers and are filled out with wheat, soya, fillers, preservatives and chemicals
- They contain dangerous levels of additives, preservatives and colourings.

However, if you are caught out with nothing to eat and you have to cheat...

- Buy one or two burgers, throw away the bread, order an extra small salad and a small portion of fries, (not Stage 1). Avoid the fizzy drinks, juices and milk shakes and order water.
- Pizza places usually do a self-serve salad bar. Avoid the salads which are drowned in mayonnaise and try and include egg and any proteins such as turkey strips or tuna. Avoid the pasta salads and potato salads. Do not have pizza.
- Buy a baked potato and pay if you need to for extra tuna or cheese filling and extra salad. The potatoes are usually huge: eat only half and include the skin, it is the most nutritious part of the potato. Avoid fried potato skins; they are full of fat and bad calories.
- One of the healthiest fast foods are shwarmas found in the Arabic cafés. I am not referring to the great fatty British kebab, which seems to attract fat as it cooks. An Arabic chicken or lamb shwarma is usually made with pure meat seasoned with Arabic spices and slowly cooked on a spit, allowing most of the fat to drip away. The meat is carved off the outside of the meat as it cooks and served in a pitta bread (better than a sandwich) with salad and sesame seed puree sauce

(tahini). It is very nutritious and a well-balanced snack. Although the pitta bread is made of wheat, it is better than burger buns. A better option is to order the Shwarma 'plate' which includes the meat, a mix of raw vegetables and salads and a carton of hummus. This is a fantastic fast food option. Do not ruin it by ordering a fruit cocktail as they contain huge amounts of fruit sugar, even if you ask them to hold on the added sugar.
- Have a single piece of fruit such as an apple or small banana after all of the above and only drink water.

Avoid
- Sandwiches
  (in desperate emergency, take the top layer of bread off a tuna, chicken or meat sandwich)
- Pasta
- Pizza
- Hot dogs
- Crispy Fried Chicken

PACKED LUNCHES

My best advice is to be prepared. Twice a week, wash and chop salad vegetables such as lettuce, chinese cabbage, rocket, baby spinach leaves, coriander, radishes, carrot, cucumber, bean sprouts, herbs, peppers, spring onions or whatever you fancy apart from tomatoes. Place enough salad for a few days in a large sealed container in the fridge. It will remain fresh without dressing for at least 4 to 5 days.

Each morning as you dash out to work, grab a couple of handfuls of your ready prepared salad and place in a smaller container, then quickly add any form of protein that you fancy that day. For example cold chicken, a tin of tuna, cold salmon or steak that you may have left over from the night before (always cook extra for the following day). You could combine some cheese chopped into cubes with some chopped cold meat or even two boiled eggs. Make your salads varied and tasty by adding lots of different ingredients.

Keep a packet of Ryvita at work and have one or two of these with your lunch. If you have access to a fridge, make up a salad dressing of olive oil and lemon juice and add it to your salad just before eating. If you are still hungry take a piece of fruit to be eaten immediately after lunch or a live plain yoghurt with a teaspoon of honey. Delicious, easy and no excuses!

If you do not fancy salad every day, though do try and ensure you eat plenty of salads and greens during the week, you could eat up to three Ryvita with protein in the form of:
- Tuna mayonnaise (use no more than 2 teaspoons of mayo for one tin of tuna)
- Egg mayonnaise
- Mozarella with basil
- Cold meat e.g. plain roast ham, turkey, chicken, beef with lettuce, mustard, little mayonnaise
- Smoked salmon and or goats cheese or a little cream cheese

Follow with a portion of fruit or a plain live yoghurt with a little honey

Hot Options
High quality ready made meals are fine if you have a microwave at work but avoid the starch in them during stage one and two. The best are casseroles, roast dinners or mild curries.

Case History: Rosacea and Broken Veins
Male, age 61, blood group A

At my wife's insistence I consulted Judy rather reluctantly, I am fit and healthy in my early sixties. I had no illusions that the severe rosacea and broken red veins which had covered my face for nearly 20 years could be helped. Doctors had repeatedly told me it was an incurable condition that had no known cause.

During the consultation my body told Judy otherwise. She had seen several previous cases all of which had cleared when the relevant food intolerances were eliminated from the diet. Mine was no different. 80% of the cause was modern wheat, 10% tropical fruits and 10% tomatoes. Considering I ate up to four bananas a day, I hadn't given myself a chance.

With strict elimination together with B12, Flax seed and the herb Butchers Broom, as prescribed by my body, the effect was dramatic. Within three weeks my nose and mid cheeks had nearly cleared of red veins. Over the next two months, it completely cleared. I am left with just a few tiny veins on my outer cheeks. These, my body tells Judy, will all disappear in time. Twice I have inadvertently cheated, once on croutons, once on a peach and within an hour, the redness had returned with a vengeance. It was gone again by the next morning.

As a bonus of being on this programme, I have dropped two notches on my belt and feel fantastic, clean inside I would describe it. Judy has developed an extraordinary ability to diagnose the underlying causes of many complexing medical conditions. This eating programme is just the beginning of many already proven discoveries.

J.N.

CHAPTER 9

SUGGESTED SUPPLEMENT PROGRAMME

Over the past four years of asking the body directly what vitamins, minerals and supplements it needs I have been surprised how much the body's requirements differ from how we normally take supplements. Time after time it prefers higher doses taken for a short period of time only. Rocket fuel to put us back into orbit so to speak. For example, the daily recommended dosage of B12 would be around two hundred and fifty to five hundred micrograms a day for several months. The body however has never requested less than one thousand but will only take it for two to three months at the most. According to our bodies, vitamins and minerals taken in supplement form in low dosages are ineffective and have little impact on our health. Over four years, I had very few cases, except in exceptional circumstances where the body is genetically deficient in a certain vitamin or mineral, or we are treating a long term condition, where long term supplementation of anything has been recommended. Booster programmes for the immune system are best taken one month on, one month off. The exception of course is before or during pregnancy where supplements should be taken for a prolonged period. If the doses are not high enough, most of the supplement is destroyed in the digestive process or eliminated by the body, as they are difficult to absorb in a non-bio form. On this programme, you will receive all the nutrition you need to be healthy. The following programme is optional and designed to boost your immune system and metabolic rate if you feel particularly sluggish at the moment. It should be taken for up to three months only, except for the turmeric which is the body's choice to break down cellulite and which must be taken for at least six months to be effective.

B12: The King of Supplements
If I had to choose just one supplement that had the greatest overall benefit, it would be this one. B12 is a water-soluble vitamin and is vital for normal metabolism of nerve tissue and is directly involved in protein, fat and carbohydrate metabolism. It aids in the production of all-important DNA and RNA, the body's genetic material and is an incredible healing accelerator. Take between 1000mcg and 2000mcg a day depending on how run down you feel. The body appears to have no problem absorbing it in capsule form. You may well be taking it because you are deficient in it, but because it will assist greatly in your detox and general well being. It is also excellent in balancing brain chemistry.

If you suspect you are intolerant to yeast, look for a yeast free brand.

Alfalfa:
This herb is nature's natural multiple vitamin supplement and because it is in a balanced bio form is much more easily absorbed and utilised by your body. Alfalfa contains nearly every mineral and vitamin you need. Take 1500mg a day for two to three months.

Selenium:
Without adequate quantities of selenium we are highly susceptible to cancer, viruses and free radical damage. It is excellent for accelerating the removal of toxins from our systems and is one of the most potent free radical scavengers that we call antioxidants. A deficiency causes poor resistance to viruses and bacteria and reduces T-cell activity. Take 200 mg daily for two to three months.

CoEnzyme Q10:
Often referred to as the spark of life, CoQ10 increases antibody production and has antiviral, antibacterial and anti-tumour effects. This is the vitamin that helps release energy from your cells and will help you through the low points of the detox! By the time we reach the age of 50, our CoQ10 level is only half what it was when we were 20. You would have to eat pounds of CoQ10 foods daily, such as sardines and peanuts, to obtain adequate levels and most of us, except the lucky A blood-types are intolerant to peanuts. Take 75mg for two to three months.

L-Glutathione:
No other antioxidant is as important to overall health as glutathione. It is the regenerator of immune cells and the most valuable detoxifying agent in the body. Low levels bring about early ageing and even death. Optimal levels make your immune cells extremely efficient. Glutathione is composed of three amino acids-cysteine, glutamic acid and glycine. It is produced in every cell of the body with the aid of selenium, magnesium and Vitamin C. It is absorbed through the gut and is important for its antioxidant activity in the gastrointestinal tract. Watermelon and avocado are the richest food sources of glutathione, the much-maligned avocado also being a valuable source of mono-unsaturated fats, which play a vital role in oxidation and the control of free radicals. If you have any bowel problems, take this supplement for up to three months. The recommended dose is 100mg daily.

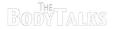

Magnesium:
If you are feeling run down and irritable, take 400mg of an easily absorbable form of magnesium called magnesium malate for two months. Magnesium is one of those wonderful minerals that helps in the absorption of many other minerals such as calcium and phosphorous but due to depletion in our soils is not as abundant as it once was. Great for enhancing and balancing moods.

Evening Primrose Oil:
Evening Primrose Oil is a rich source of fat burning gamma linolenic acid. As well as balancing hormones it helps flush the body of stubborn fats. Take a 500mg capsule daily.

Potassium:
Potassium helps regulate water balance within the body by regulating the distribution of fluids on either side of the cell walls and as a result helps control water retention and bloating. It is vital for the takeup of the thyroid hormones by the cells. Take one 99mg tablet daily for three months.

Cayenne Pepper:
This spice is excellent for boosting your metabolic rate and if you cannot find it in capsule form, can be bought as a fresh spice from the supermarket. Take 500mg a day or half a teaspoon of fresh spice mixed with some yoghurt.

Turmeric:
The body has told me that this herb is fantastic for clearing CELLULITE!! Take 1500mg a day in capsule form or one and a half teaspoons of fresh powder for a minimum of 6 months to increase circulation and flush out the toxins.

Supplements are best taken after breakfast.

TIP: Cellulite is not caused by fat. It is a combination of food intolerances, chemical toxins and hormones which become trapped in the fat cells. The Cellular Detox, regular skin brushing with a natural bristle brush and ten minutes a day bouncing on a mini trampoline, will eventually help remove this orange peel horror from which most women suffer. And I mean eventually! It may take months.

IF YOU SUFFER WITH SUGAR CRAVINGS…

Chromium:
Chromium stimulates the activity of enzymes involved in the metabolism of glucose for energy and the synthesis of fatty acids and cholesterol. It increases the effectiveness of insulin, preventing hypoglycaemia (too much insulin) and diabetes (too little insulin). Take 200mcg daily.

L-Glutamine:
This amino acid can reach a brain starved of sugar and craving for a fix within minutes and immediately feed the body's need for glucose. It is a natural food substance which stabilizes our mental function and promotes good digestion. It is an amazing supplement if you are addicted to carbohydrates. It will be of huge help in the early days of this programme if you have become dependent on carbohydrates to feel full. Take 4 x 500mg a day, 2 on rising before breakfast and 2 mid afternoon to kick in for that late afternoon sweet craving. It should always be taken on an empty stomach with water.

P.S. If you want to give up smoking, use this amazing supplement to help with the cravings. Take up to 10 x 500mg quite safely, 2 every few hours between meals in the first month that you stop. It will make all the difference.

L-Tyrosine:
This amino acid will stimulate the thyroid if you suspect yours is sluggish and lift tiredness within minutes of taking it. Take 1-2 capsules of 500mg a day, one on rising and one mid afternoon. Take with water on an empty stomach. Do not take if you are under medication for your thyroid.

TABLE OF SUPPLEMENTS

Supplement	Daily amount	When to take it
B12	1000-2000mcg	After breakfast
Alfalfa	1500mg	After breakfast
Selenium	200mg	After breakfast
CoQ10	75mg	After breakfast
Magnesium	400mg	After breakfast
Glutathione	100mg	After breakfast
Evening Primrose Oil	500mg	At bedtime
Potassium	99mg	After breakfast
Cayenne Pepper	500mg	After breakfast
Turmeric	1500mg	After breakfast

For Sugar Cravings...

Supplement	Daily amount	When to take it
Chromium	200mcg	After breakfast
L-Glutamine	1000mg	500mg on rising/500mg mid afternoon

Optional for lethargy and/or sluggish thyroid

Supplement	Daily amount	When to take it
L-Tyrosine	500-1000mg	500mg on rising/500mg mid afternoon

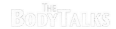

Case History: Graves Disease or Hyperthyroidism
Jackie, 42 years old, blood group O

Jackie came to see me complaining of severe bloating, constipation and discomfort after eating. She mentioned that she had a long-term overactive thyroid, and had been taking medication for this condition for the past two years. As conventional medicine does not understand why it is that the thyroid becomes over or under-active, it is thought to be incurable and sufferers are expected to take medication for life. Jackie felt that the medication was not proving effective, but she had come to accept that this was the best she could feel. Unusually for someone diagnosed as suffering from Hyperthyroidism, she was overweight and exhibited signs of significant fluid retention.

During her consultation, Jackie's body told me that she had Candida Albicans. Muscle testing also revealed that classic O blood type food intolerances (including wheat, coffee and tea) were affecting her thyroid.

Following two months of strict elimination of food intolerances, a course of supplements prescribed by her body and a further five months of careful diet, Jackie's thyroid normalised, and she has been able to come off all medication. Limiting her intake of food intolerances has kept Jackie's thyroid stable for the past 3 years.

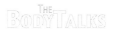

CHAPTER 10

FOOD TIPS AND USEFUL INFORMATION

Aspartame (Nutrasweet, Equal, Spoonful etc)
Very nasty and very poisonous. When the temperature of aspartame exceeds 86 degrees F. the wood alcohol in aspartame converts to formaldehyde and then to formic acid, which in turn causes metabolic acidosis and changes the brain's chemistry. The methanol toxicity mimics multiple sclerosis, thus many people are being wrongly diagnosed. Multiple Sclerosis is not a death sentence, whereas methanol toxicity is. Three to four 12oz cans of diet soda a day can trigger systemic lupus or multiple sclerosis symptoms. Aspartame makes you crave carbohydrates and makes you fat and I have seen people lose up to 20 pounds just coming off the diet soda and sweeteners. Aspartame is particularly deadly for diabetics. Avoid all 'diet', 'low sugar' or 'sugar free' foods, which contain it. (See Excitotoxins: The Taste that Kills by Dr. Russell Blaylock (Heath Press 1-800-643-2665)

Almonds
The prince of nuts, nature's perfectly balanced highly nutritious snack. Best eaten plain or roasted, not salted. Contain equal amounts of protein and carbohydrate and a high level of good Omega 3 unsaturated fats. Their saturated fat content is only 10%. They are high in calories, which makes them ideal to make up your calorie allowance on a low starch diet but fattening if you eat too many. Limit a snack serving to a maximum of eight to ten nuts. They are chock full of calcium, magnesium and potassium. Cashew nuts are also similar, eat in small snack sizes of up to 8 nuts. A handful of 8 nuts a day will supply all your calcium needs to keep your bones healthy in a bioabsorpable form and is much more effective than taking a calcium suppliment.

Avocados
This wonderful fruit is an excellent source of good fat and cholesterol and is full of digestive enzymes. Although high in calories, in terms of nutrients per calorie they are a Superfood and two or three avocados a week in your salads are a great source of folic acid, B vitamins and potassium. They are an excellent source of dietary cholesterol,... enjoy them!

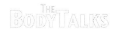

Butter

A natural good saturated fat when eaten in moderation. Butter is an excellent food, full of nutrients and the shorter fats that are easiest for us to digest and burn as fuel. Even most lactose intolerant A Blood types can tolerate butter. The best alternatives available on the market are soft spreads made with olive oil. I have not found one other margarine on the market that the body has not consistently tested negatively with including all the major brands. Our bodies have evolved with butter over many years, do not be afraid to use it. Your body needs some natural saturated fats and it is far better to eat natural fats than man made ones. Butter is also the only fat which does not change its molecular structure when heated. As explained in The Body Talks Programme, all oils become dangerous and poisonous when heated and should not be used for any cooking. Ignore all the marketing on the benefits of cooking with oil, even olive oil. Return to nature and use a little butter. Your palate will love it and your heart will not suffer, quite the contrary.

Bread

The two main components of bread are wheat and yeast, two of the most common food intolerances. If you are yeast intolerant, then all wheat free breads can also give you problems. My tests of over 2000 people show that around 98% of us are intolerant to modern day hybrid wheat, a form of wheat modified from original Spelt wheat over the last 130 years, through selective breeding and genetic modification. Wheat free breads, made with 100% rye flour or old-fashioned Spelt flour are becoming more readily available in health food shops and supermarkets. Also keep in mind that one slice of bread contains around 18 grams of starch carbohydrate. Most people need only around 30 grams of starch in the whole day. As Cindy Crawford is famously quoted as saying "You may as well just sit on it". Bread is fattening, period. If you are trying to lose weight, substitute Ryvita for bread and eat lots of low carbohydrate nutritious vegetables. Consign regular bread consumption to the past. Unless you are very physically active, eating bread will make weight control an ongoing battle.

Coffee

The 'O' and 'B' blood groups are intolerant to a protein in the coffee bean, not the caffeine. They may also be caffeine intolerant but that is separate, hence decaffeinated coffee is not the answer. If you are a heavy coffee drinker of around five or more cups a day, cut down slowly over the first week and then go cold turkey. If you drink under five cups a day, cut it out immediately. You will suffer from a couple of days of bad headaches, but drink lots of water and take a mild painkiller if desperate. The idea is to trigger a cellular clean out from the cells of old coffee toxic residue, which cannot happen if you are drinking even one coffee every five days. The 'A' blood type actually likes and thrives on coffee but limit your intake to no more than three a day, without milk of course and with only one sugar maximum. Try cream or goat's milk instead of cow's milk.

Coffee alternatives are limited to dandelion coffee and chicory, the latter of which may also be a food intolerance for some people. Your taste buds are your best guide.

Chemicals
We live in a chemical world. Chemicals have played a major role both in increasing our standard of living in the last 100 years and in destroying our precious planet and our health. Levels of chemical residue in our bodies are now alarmingly high, to the extent that corpses are now decomposing much slower! Cancer will continue to increase to epidemic proportions, I fear, until we recognise the part chemicals play in inducing it.

Meanwhile, you can help yourself by becoming aware of where they are to be found in the highest concentrations. Many people are unaware of the chemicals used in skin lotions, shampoos, body products, detergents and household cleaners. We use these products daily and tiny amounts of chemicals are being absorbed through the skin or inhaled each day, slowly building up to a toxic level in our bodies. All of these products, including some of the more expensive beauty products and creams, come up regularly as a major contributing cause in allergies, skin disorders and rashes, eczema, aches and pains, headaches and as a contributing factor to cancer. Switch to natural products, especially for skin and hair products, and where possible, household detergents, particularly washing-up liquid. Ask in your local health food shop for natural alternatives. The best shampoo I have found that is easily available and has little allergy reaction for most people, although it does contain SLS, is the Body Shop Ginger Shampoo. Please never discontinue this wonderful product Body Shop!

Deodorants can be particularly harmful as they are absorbed through the underarms into the lymphatic system and repeated use builds up toxic residue. The body has cited this buildup as a cause of breast cancer, as the body, in its infinite wisdom, attempts to channel the toxins away from vital organs to an area that even if removed, does not ultimately threaten life. In this instance, breast cancer may be a bet-

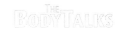

ter option, but prevention is much, much better than the cure. Avoid chemical deodorants and use natural crystal, aluminium free or herbal products.

Chemicals in foods are also on the increase as foods need to have a longer shelf life or have extra flavourings and colourings added to meet an ever-increasing taste for more salty, sugary, stronger flavoured food. By reading labels and becoming aware of what is added to foods, you will be able to make the best choices available to you with what you are offered. Ideally, cook for yourself using raw natural products but we will never be able to avoid all chemicals; it is possibly too late for that in the current world, but vote with your feet and buy organic or natural whenever you can. Become a conscious consumer; do not believe anything you read about new man-made foods or products that stand to make multinationals big profits. Become knowledgeable about the way food is produced. It may save your life. It will help the future of our planet and the choices our children have to eat natural food.

Chicken
Every 'B' Blood type I have tested and about 10% of 'A' blood types are highly intolerant to chicken. According to Dr Peter D'Adamo, author of the best selling "Eat Right For Your Type". A protein in chicken causes severe blood clotting in the 'B' blood group which highly increases your chances of a stroke. Chicken was the major cause of my multiple sclerosis symptoms and that of many other sufferers of this debilitating disease, according to their bodies when I have asked them. I made a full recovery after four years and other sufferers are feeling better since eliminating it from their diet. I only have to eat it twice in a week for the numbness to reoccur in my left toes.

The intensive farming methods of producing chicken has led to very high use of antibiotics and hormones in the feed, which naturally get passed into the bird and subsequently on to us. This is definitely one meat where free range or organic is worth the price if you eat a lot of it. Turkey is a better option. It is similar to chicken in most respects but does not contain the dangerous proteins. They are also quite intensively farmed however, and also contain antibiotics and hormones.

Constipation
This is possibly one of the hardest conditions I treat. And one of the most common. Frequent underlying causes I have found through asking the body are bacteria in the large intestine, food intolerances and par-

asites. Unfortunately, even once the cause is eliminated, the damage done over many years leaves the natural peristaltic movement of the intestine, which moves the food through the body, weakened and lazy. It takes on average a minimum of five months to achieve any kind of normal bowel movement in most cases.

In total opposition to the established rule that constipation should be treated with extra fibre, particularly bran and raw veggies, the body repeatedly requests that you reduce the intake of raw fibre if the bowels are blocked and eat more soft baby type foods such as well cooked vegetables, soft fruits, yoghurt, soups and such. A large bowl of cooked vegetables daily is full of fibre but is easy to digest. If there is inflammation or irritable bowel syndrome present, which is the case nine times out of ten, the fibre found in whole grains, raw salads, raw vegetables and unpeeled fruits, can act like a scouring pad against the raw flesh, aggravating a very sensitive intestinal wall. Many cases of food intolerance related constipation are entirely due to our old friend, modern hybrid wheat. Often just avoiding foods containing wheat gives rapid relief. The results of this low fibre approach speak for themselves. Wheat is also a major cause of haemorrhoids, which magically clear up after a few months when wheat is eliminated from the diet. Try it, it may work for you. The Body Talks programme includes plenty of good fibre in your diet to maintain a healthy bowel function as long as you are eating plenty of salads, vegetables, nuts and seeds. Regular exercise and plenty of water are essential for healthy bowels.

The best natural laxative is a natural form of fibre called psillium husks, found in health shops. Alternatively try linseeds: a teaspoon or more mixed with plain, live yoghurt is an easy way to take them. Seneca from the pharmacy is also natural but like all laxatives will become less and less effective if used too often.

A less common but distressing detox symptom of avoiding your food intolerances is the development of constipation. Unbeknown to you, your food intolerance may have had a loosening affect on your bowels over many years, causing the natural bowel peristaltic movement of the small and large intestine to become lazy. When these foods are naturally eliminated that diarrhoea affect is removed, and the lazy bowels may take several weeks to six months to begin to work normally. **Do not add fibre**, by resorting to softer, well cooked vegetables and fruit, the weakened bowel will slowly recover. Psillium husks and/or senecca will aid the movement. Drink plenty of water and be patient. The opposite affect often occurs if you have suffered with constipation before you start the elimination. Food intolerances, particularly wheat, can paralyse the gut but it quickly begins to work once the culprits are avoided

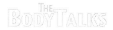

Cream

Cream is the fat content of milk and as long as it is pure cream, not half and half, does not contain significant levels of either protein or lactose, making it tolerable in moderation for most people who are intolerant to milk. As cream is a fat, it can only be turned to body fat when eaten with sugars, for example cream and fruit, or cream and pasta. When eaten with protein or very low starch vegetables it is fine. It makes a useful base for meat sauces or to thicken vegetable soups such as broccoli or mushroom without being converted to body fat. Eat bread with the soup, however, and a different story ensues as the insulin is released in response to the carbohydrate, which then traps the cream as body fat in your cells. Remember, it is very high in saturated fat, calories and cholesterol and should be used respectfully and moderately.

Diet foods and drinks

This refers to all foods and drinks labelled sugar free, diet, low or no fat or cholesterol free or diabetic. They are all man made, unnatural, deceptive, hide chemicals and poisonous substitute substances such as aspartame or transfatty acids and should be avoided, all of them, at all costs. I have not found one that the body says is good for it or really delivers on its promise. Someone has to say it!! The industry is worth billions because we have fallen for the marketing. These products are not researched by independent scientists: they are developed by the scientists who work for the food company which stands to make millions from a successful, new food, marketed and backed up by their research. Call me cynical. Ulltimately, regular use of any of these products will lead to accelerated metabolic ageing and an unbalanced immune system.

Eggs

Eggs are nature's wonder food and THE best food for weight loss and maintaining sugar levels. They contain a superb balance of chromium, lecithin, B vitamins, good cholesterol, fats and protein. 94% of the protein in egg is used by the body compared to only 34% of the protein in meat. Eggs do not cause high cholesterol, they actually lower it. In 1999, a study on 100,000 people in the USA looked at the relationship between egg consumption and raised cholesterol levels. There was no significant link. Eggs actually can lower cholesterol if cholesterol levels are high. Two eggs a day will convince the body it is receiving enough vital dietary cholesterol and that it can switch off the enzyme ADH reductase in the liver, whose sole job it is to manufacture extra cholesterol from incoming sugars. There is not one study that links eggs to high cholesterol and heart disease. It is an assumed relationship because eggs are high in cholesterol. In the last three years I have had 28 cases of high cholesterol, non of which were responding to normal low cholesterol diets or drugs. They returned to normal cholesterol levels within three to four months after eating two eggs a day.

Eggs can cause constipation when hard-boiled in their shells. The shell, which gives the unique toughness to the egg is released during cooking into the egg, which causes binding in the intestines. An occasional hard boiled egg is fine, but cook eggs out of their shells if you are prone to constipation. Eggs make the best breakfast. Try and buy eggs of good quality, preferably free range or corn fed with a low level of hormone or antibiotic. A fresh egg will sink when placed in water, whereas an older egg will have absorbed air through the shell and will float.

In April 1999 a study published in the Journal of American Medical Association of over 100,000 subjects, found no correlation between the daily consumption of eggs and the incidence of heart disease or strokes in men and women.

Frying
Frying in ANY oil including olive oil causes short-term memory loss according to the body as heated oils change their molecular structure and become very toxic. Heating to high temperatures such as those reached during frying, damages fat, which cannot be recognised by the body and broken down and properly digested and eliminated. These then become cellular toxic waste, which directly affects the brain and damages cells by clogging them up. The accumulated debris causes accelerated ageing and contributes to furring up of arteries. Any unnatural man made fat, such as sunflower and corn oils, margarines and other low fat spreads which are also damaged fats do the same thing. The body has recommended we fry in butter or ghee, not a lot and not often, but as these are saturated fats, they remain stable in a safe digestible form at high temperatures.

Genetically Engineered Foods
Genetically engineered foods contain genes from other plants and animals, introduced to give them certain qualities such as a higher yield, a certain flavour or resistance to certain pests. The problem is there have been no long-term human safety tests done on the consumption of these foods, nor do we really know the impact that they may have on our natural world.

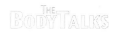

Initial evidence is very worrying and is showing strong warning signs of its massive impact on the future of our environment and our health. Genetic pollution from pollen drift is spreading widely outside the test growth areas, costing millions in lost export sales. In Iowa, in North America, corn farmers planted 1% of their crop in GE "Starlink" seed, not approved for human consumption. Within 12 months, 50% of the entire Iowa corn crop tested positive for traces of the Starlink gene, according to David Gould of Farm Verified Organic. Super weeds, resistant to known herbicides, are appearing in areas planted with GM seeds containing a herbicide resistant gene.

The worrying increase of asthma in Britain has exactly mirrored the increase in imports of genetically engineered soy being imported from America.

For those of us intolerant to certain natural foods, the implications of GM foods are terrifying. You will not know if you are eating a food which contains an element of something that makes you ill. If it takes the human body so many years (around 10-20 generations) to become tolerant to a new natural food, what will be the damage to our health on a global level with the introduction of GM foods? There is also no room for experimentation here. Once these pollens are released, we can never go back.

Gluten
Gluten is a protein found in most grains such as wheat, oats, barley and rye. Corn, rice and millet do not contain gluten. Gluten is a protein that in some people attacks the lining of the stomach and causes inflammation and even ulceration of the delicate digestive tract. In some cases the gluten protein interferes directly with the brain or delicate membranes throughout the body, such as in the joints or sinuses. A true gluten allergy is quite rare, occurring in only 1 in 250 people I test. This condition is known medically as Coeliac disease and can be very serious. It is closely associated with both diabetes and colon cancer. If you are wheat intolerant it does not mean you are gluten intolerant. Most people are intolerant to the modifications in the make up of modern day wheat, not to the gluten. Gluten free breads and biscuits are automatically wheat free and can be used in a wheat free diet, but are not necessary. People with gluten allergies can only eat gluten free starches, such as corn, rice, potato, quinoa, millet, maize and kamut.

Saliva, Blood, Skin Prick, or Biopsy for Severe Gluten Intolerances (Coeliac Disease)
If you suspect you have a gluten allergy, the gold standard for hormone testing according to the World Health Organisation is a saliva test, which seems to identify it reliably from mild to severe. The blood

test only seems to identify the most severe coeliac cases. Specialised skin-prick testing is another reliable allergy test, but the most accurate way of diagnosing true coeliac disease is by biopsy of the small intestine. The body will tell me the level of intolerance or allergy to gluten by a percentage value, but when I suspect a gluten allergy I always ask people to get a medical test to confirm this.

Gluten intolerance is a much milder form of this reaction, which many people may suffer. Grains are generally difficult to digest and I do not advise anyone to eat too many of them. The phytic acid found in grains is also known to block the absorption of calcium. Grains are also a starch form of carbohydrate and contain high amounts of concentrated sugars. Common gluten intolerance symptoms, usually only felt with the higher levels of gluten found in modern day wheat, include bloating, gas, low energy, fluid retention, cellulite and even sleepiness.

Modern day wheat is the result of 150 years of selective breeding and hybridisation and is approximately three times higher in gluten than original spelt wheat. Rye, barley and oats are still fairly close to their original natural form and have been, in their current form, in the human diet for hundreds of years. It is not known exactly how the changes from original spelt into new modern wheat have affected us, but there is no doubt that an increasing number of people today are suffering adverse effects in some way from it. 94% of the 2000 people I have tested to date were intolerant to modern wheat, not gluten and were able to eat original spelt wheat, rye, barley and oats.

Goat's milk
Goat's milk is lactose free and ideal for those unable to take dairy foods. It is nutritious and balanced and is a much better substitute for dairy than soya milk, particularly in infants. It is now readily available in most countries in supermarkets and can be used for drinking and cooking. It is stronger tasting than cow's milk and not to everyone's taste. Available in semi skimmed in many countries.

Herbal Teas
If you are an O, B or AB blood type, coffee and black tea, such as breakfast, Earl Grey, Darjeeling for example, will not be good for you, whether or not you are intolerant to caffeine. Therefore decaffeinated tea or coffee is not better for you. There are however good substitutes for both which also have health benefits that coffee and black tea do not have. (See list on following page).

The following teas are good for....

Tea	Good for...
Aniseed	Boosting the immune system
Camomile	Relieving upset stomachs, colds and fevers in children. A sleep inducer and mild sedative
Dandelion	Tastes more like coffee. Excellent for the absorption of iron
Fennel and Nettle	Cleansing the kidneys and detoxifying the blood
Ginger	Increases stomach acid secretion, very good digestive, especially for the A and AB blood types
Ginseng	Has a positive effect on the nervous system, particularly for the B blood type
Goldenseal	Indigestion and liver disorders. A natural laxative and diuretic. Weak tea help to relieve nausea during pregnancy
Peppermint	Tummy ache and digestive bloating and gas. Stimulates digestive secretions
Rooibos or Redbush	A South African tea which tastes and brews similar to black tea. Has excellent antioxidant and general health tonic properties. Caffeine free and very low in tannin
Rose Hips	A good kidney and bladder tonic. Very high in vitamin C and helpful in preventing colds
Sarsaparilla	Boosting the immune system and can kill some viruses. Excellent blood purifier and detoxification tea
Thyme (Zatar)	A good immune booster and tonic for the throat and voice

Honey

Honey is a natural sugar and is a better sweetener than either sugar or chemical substitutes. It is still however a form of sugar and will trigger insulin in the blood. Use sparingly to sweeten plain yoghurt and herbal teas. A teaspoon of honey a day, grown in your home area of about five miles, may help combat hay fever during the summer. Because the bees have gathered the pollen from the grasses and plants that are causing your symptoms, the honey acts as a vaccine against them, often reducing your reaction. It will need to be taken for at least three months for the effect to be felt.

Ice cream

If you are lactose intolerant, many people can still tolerate real ice cream, made with cream, as the cream is the fat of the milk and contains no lactose. Go for the really good makes such as Ben and Jerry's and Haagen Das, which do not contain any milk but are made with pure cream. Beware the sugar in ice cream and eat it after a meal to slow down the digestion of the sugar. Good ice-cream substitutes for those who are very sensitive to lactose include frozen yoghurts (the lactose in yoghurt is broken down by the live bacteria), sorbets and the occasional soy ice cream which, if eaten rarely, will not have any detrimental effects on your body.

Menopause

I have over 150 women clients currently taking natural Hormone Replacement Therapy (HRT) in the form of Wild Yam, Dong Quai and Black Cohosh capsules. These natural herb substitutes for low progesterone and oestrogen have no side effects and are used by the body as required, meaning any excess is eliminated if not needed. All the women in full menopause are taking 1500mg daily of Wild Yam to replace the progesterone and *either* 80mg of Dong Quai *or* Black Cohosh, well above the current recommended doses which are not strong enough to have any effect. Women who have tried the herbs but have not taken enough therefore think they don't work, and as a result, have not seen the incredible benefits of these herbs. To date, very few, if any, full studies have been carried out on natural HRT and a required dosage has never been established properly. The body has repeatedly insisted on this dosage in my clients and the benefits have been wonderful with no reported adverse effects. The last two herbs must not be taken together as the body says they cancel each other out. You will either be a Dong Quai or a Black Cohosh person, never both. Without personal testing I would recommend you begin the programme with Wild Yam and Dong Quai only at first. If Don Quai is right for you, you will feel much bet-

ter within three weeks. If you feel no real improvement or even a worsening of your symptoms, continue the Wild Yam but stop the Dong Quai. Wait three days and then start the Black Cohosh. One of them will work wonders for 99% of you. I have only had 2 ladies whose bodies have actually preferred the chemical HRT. When we tried the cream options, most women found them to be less effective and prefer the capsules. Sage Tea is also excellent for stopping hot flushes. Women beginning menopause can take half the above dose for the first year at the first sign of symptoms. This programme is highly effective in preventing all the downfalls of menopause such as loss of bone density, hair and muscle loss and dryness. The herbs can be continued over all the menopausal years without any fear of side effects.
I would also not recommend using soya products unless you have Japanese, Chinese or South American ancestry. Please see the entry on Soya for more information.

Oranges

Surprisingly, oranges are one of the most common food intolerances in all the blood types. The orange turns acidic when it is in the stomach whereas the lemon and lime become alkaline during digestion. The O blood type in particular finds oranges very acidic and they are a common cause of heartburn and discomfort but also occur frequently as a contributing food causing arthritis and joint ache. My advice in the light of the huge percentage of my clients I have tested who cannot tolerate oranges (around 80%) is to switch to less acidic citrus fruit like grapefruit or to other juices such as pineapple. A general good rule to follow is to always water down juices by at least half. This will halve the amount of sugar and calories that are contained in freshly squeezed and concentrated fruit juices. Lemon and lime will neutralize acidity in the stomach and are excellent digestives. Squeeze $\frac{1}{2}$ into a cup of water to cleanse the system first thing in the morning or after a meal if you are prone to indigestion.

Rice

Like bread, when it comes to rice, you may as well sit on it. It will very quickly put excess pounds on your tummy and thighs. White rice is very fattening! All the goodness and fibre is removed from brown rice when it is refined into white rice. It is high in starch and low in nutrients. Two tablespoons of cooked white rice equals around thirty grams of carbohydrate or six teaspoons of white sugar. More often we will eat a minimum of four tablespoons of rice at a meal. Try and limit your rice intake at a meal to just one to two tablespoons of white rice or two to three of brown. Always combine it with some fat, protein and vegetables to try and slow down the digestion of the sugar.

Brown rice contains four times the fibre and approximately two times the nutrients of white rice. Even though a cup of brown and white rice contain the same number of calories, the fibre in the brown rice slows down its digestion and the sugar is released into the blood more slowly, making it less likely to be turned to body fat. Wild rice is a seed, not a grain and contains much higher levels of protein and 25% less carbohydrate and calories. It needs to be cooked for at least an hour until the seed bursts and opens out into a soft delicious food. Add a little fried onion, peppers, peas and corn for an excellent side dish to accompany any meal. Limit your portion to 2 tablespoons.

Soya
Unless you have inherited Japanese or South American genetics, beware of soya and all soy products. This is a new food only introduced to the west in the last 20 years and 99% of western people I test for soy are highly intolerant to it. Your body has not been able to adjust and evolve into the very high level of natural hormones contained in this food. The 1% of westerners that I found could take soy all had some Japanese or South American ancestry, cultures which have eaten soya for centuries.

In 1999, two top scientists, working for the Food and Drug Administration in America, broke rank with their colleagues and wrote an internal protest letter, opposing the FDA's decision to approve a health claim that soya reduced the risk of heart disease. They warned of 28 studies disclosing the toxic effects of soya, revealing their studies had all produced significant and dangerous levels of breast cancer, brain damage and abnormalities in infants. In an interview with the Observer newspaper in the UK in August 1999, one of the soya experts, Daniel Doerge, said: 'Research has shown a clear link between soya and the potential for adverse effects in humans.' These studies were carried out on a western population. The studies that support the widely publicised benefits of taking soy, all result from longitudinal studies on people whose cultures have eaten soy products as a main part of their diets for hundreds of years. Yes, for them soy is beneficial and can protect against cancer. But for the westerner, the opposite is true. It is not just in vegetarian products such as tofu and soya milk that the danger lies. Soya is a key ingredient in products from meat sausages and fish fingers to salad creams and breakfast cereals. The soya industry, worth six billion dollars in the States each year alone, insists that the health benefits outweigh the risks. Richard Barnes, European director of the US Soy Bean Association said: "Millions of people around the world have been eating soya for years and have shown no signs of abnormalities". Have we? It is difficult to prove my claim unless scientific tests are made public, but having tested so many people for soya

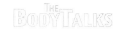

and had it rejected 100% of the time, I am not convinced it is safe for Westerners with no history of soya in their cultures. Add to this the fact so much of it is now genetically modified. I strongly advise you avoid all soya productsuntil more is known about the long-term effects it may have on us, if we are ever going to be told the truth. This includes soy milk, tofu, soy sauce unless used very occasionally and soybeans. If you are vegetarian, use other seeds, nuts and pulses which are also high in protein and much safer.

Further studies have also indicated that a chemical found in soya may damage the sexual organs of boys in the womb and make them less fertile as adults. Pregnant women who eat soy could therefore be endangering their babies. A British scientific advisory panel warned that there is 'clear evidence' of a potential risk from soy-based formula milk for babies. The findings may help explain the growing incidence of infertility problems. The average sperm count of European males has dropped by a quarter in 25 years, and one in six couples in Britain now has difficulty conceiving.

Spelt
Spelt is original wheat, before it was selectively bred and modified into modern wheat. It contains approximately only a third of the gluten found in modern wheat and is highly digestible. Most people who are intolerant to wheat can eat spelt. A staple in biblical times, spelt makes a tasty nutty bread, which though heavier than modern bread due to the low gluten content, can be bought in specialist bakeries or made at home. It makes a delicious though crumbly pastry and is a good substitute in cakes and biscuits. It requires less water in recipes due to the lower gluten content. It is of course still starch and should be eaten in moderation. One slice of wholemeal spelt bread contains 15 to 18grams of carbohydrate, although it is high in fibre and highly nutritious.

Tea (see also herbal tea)
Black tea tests negatively for 99% of O and B blood type clients that I test. Black teas include Breakfast tea, Earl Gray, Darjeeling, Indian tea, etc. It is not the caffeine but something in the protein of the tea leaf and the processing of black teas that these blood types strongly object to. For these blood types it is very toxic and I have observed that even one cup of tea a day, is enough to stop many of the O and B clients reaching full health. Try Rooibos tea, a tea from a different bush grown only in South Africa which tastes and brews very similarly to black tea, but contains no caffeine and is very low in tannin. It is high in antioxidants and is growing in popularity around the world for its health giving properties. It is sold as

Rooibos or Red Bush tea in health shops all over the world. Many supermarkets now stock it as do some forward thinking hotels and restaurants. Green tea and herbal teas are also excellent.

Wheat
My experience with wheat personally and in the multitude of health problems it causes in hundreds of my clients prompts me to state that I believe modern day wheat to be responsible for many health problems today. These include diabetes, irritable bowel problems, constipation, migraines and headaches, back problems, heart attacks, strokes, allergies, ADDH and hormonal imbalances to name a few common ones. Wheat feeds viruses and damages the immune system in around 90% of my clients.

In the late 1860's, man began to selectively breed wheat to increase the yield of the crop. They took the original wheat grain we now call Spelt, and through cross-pollination increased the size of the germ twofold and in doing so doubled the gluten content. The gluten is the part of the wheat that causes the springiness and chewiness of modern day breads. However, before long, the new grains became more and more susceptible to attack by bugs and fungus and it became necessary to increase the toughness of the husk surrounding the germ to protect it. That husk is now as tough as PVC and even hydrochloric acid struggles to dissolve it. Our digestive systems also struggle and very few people seem to be able to digest it easily without any impact on either the digestive tract or immune system. Modern day wheat is a completely different grain than the ancient wheat grain of our ancestors. It is also our staple diet and we eat far more than our bodies can digest and detoxify from. Spelt flour is now grown in a few specialised farms in the UK, Germany and Canada and is becoming more and more readily available for home baking.

Problems that have disappeared when wheat has been eliminated from the diets of my clients (for a minimum of two months) have included bloating, reflux, gas, headaches, urticaria, acne, joint pain, arthritis, sinus pain, rhinitis, dandruff, fatigue, itchiness, muscle injuries, back pain, haemorrhoids, inflammation in the joints and tightness in the chest. Of the eight people I have talked to who had survived a heart attack, the body reported wheat as 80% of the direct cause in five of them. When they eliminated wheat, further tests done three months later showed that the arteries were less furred up. In one patient who was 70 years old, the furring up of his heart arteries opened up from 80% down to 20% over a year, as confirmed by medical tests. The impact of modern day wheat on health needs to be seriously researched.

Yoghurt

Yoghurt is made when live cultures of bacteria are added to milk to curdle it. The harmless bacteria, commonly known as acidophilus and bifidus, break down the sugars known as lactose in milk and turn them into lactic acid which then curdles the fresh milk to make yoghurt. Because the lactose is broken down, live yoghurt can be eaten by anyone intolerant to the lactose in milk and eaten without any problem. To ensure complete digestion, the yoghurt should still contain live bacteria, which should be labelled on the carton. Most yoghurts which have had sugar and fruit added to them or are long-life, will no longer be live and are less beneficial to the gut. These good bacteria are vital for good colon health and for the complete breakdown of foods. A vital vitamin, vitamin K, is manufactured for the body by acidophilus and bifidus and it is a good idea to regularly eat live yoghurt or take an acidophilus supplement from time to time to ensure that there is sufficient good bacteria in your digestive tract. The bodies of several women suffering with fibroids told me that the cause of these incurable growths was a lack of vitamin K. When they took acidophilus for a year, their fibroids shrank and disappeared, without the need for any surgery or medical intervention. Every case of fibroids I have treated has responded to this intervention. A lack of vitamin K also appears to increase the production of scar tissue and adhesions in the body, and acidophilus and extra live plain yoghurt should be taken before and after any operation, for several months to reduce both these side effects of damage to tissue.

Zzzzzzz's

Optimum sleep is a luxury in our busy lives but just as getting enough is vital, getting too much can also be detrimental. However, when you are toxic, your body will automatically need more in order to spend more time trying to detoxify the build up during the day. As you go through this programme, you will find you have days of needing far more sleep as the body tries to knock you out in order to heal more deeply. As you heal you will find that you need less and less sleep as time goes by. Rather than go to bed late and wake up by an alarm, go to bed earlier during the programme and allow your body to wake you when you have had enough rest. You may be surprised at how you soon begin to wake early before the alarm. It is common to have days of feeling almost drugged with tiredness in the first few weeks of detox. A toxic system will need 8-9 hours of sleep to recover. A clean body should only need $6\frac{1}{2}$ to 7, depending of course on your activity level during the day.

CHAPTER 11

LIVER CLEANSE

Cleansing the liver of gallstones dramatically improves digestion, which is the whole basis of your health. You can expect your allergies to disappear, too, more with each cleanse you do! Incredibly, it also eliminates shoulder, upper arm and upper back pain. You have more energy and increased sense of well being.

"Cleaning the liver bile ducts is the most powerful procedure that you can do to improve your body's health".

It is the job of the liver to make bile, 2 to 3 litres in the day! The liver is full of tubes (biliary tubing) that deliver the bile to one large tube (the common bile duct). The gallbladder is attached to the common bile duct and acts as a storage reservoir. Eating fat or protein triggers the gallbladder to squeeze itself empty after about twenty minutes, and the stored bile finishes its trip down the common bile duct to the intestine.

For many people, including children, the biliary tubing is choked with gallstones. Some develop allergies or hives but some have no symptoms. When the gallbladder is scanned or X-rayed nothing is seen. Typically, they are not in the gallbladder. Not only that, most are too small and not calcified, a prerequisite for visibility on X-ray. There are over half a dozen varieties of gallstones, most of which have cholesterol crystals in them. They can be black, red, white, green or tan coloured. The green ones get their colour from being coated with bile. Other stones are composites made of many smaller ones.

As the stones grow and become more numerous the back pressure on the liver causes it to make less bile. Imagine the situation if your garden hose had marbles in it. Much less water would flow, which in turn would decrease the ability of the hose to squirt out the marbles.
With gallstones, much less cholesterol leaves the body and cholesterol levels may rise.

Gallstones, being porous, can pick up all the bacteria, cysts, viruses and parasites that are passing through the liver. In this way 'nests' of infection are formed, forever supplying the body with fresh bacteria. No stomach infection such as ulcers or intestinal bloating can be cured permanently without removing these gallstones from the liver.

CLEANSE YOUR LIVER TWICE A YEAR

Choose a day like Saturday for the cleanse, since you will be able to rest the next day.

Take **no** medicines, vitamins or pills that you can do without; they could prevent success.
Eat a **no-fat** breakfast and lunch such as cooked cereal with fruit, fruit juice, bread and preserves or honey (no butter or milk), baked potato or other vegetables with salt only. This allows the bile to build up and develop pressure in the liver. Higher pressure pushes out more stones.

Ingredients

Epsom Salts	4 tablespoons
Olive oil	Half cup (light olive oil is easier to get down)
Fresh pink grapefruit	1 large or 2 small, enough to squeeze $2/3$ to $3/4$ cup juice
Ornithine	4 to 8, tablets to be sure you can sleep. Don't skip this or you may have the worst night of your life!
Large plastic straw	To help you drink the mixture
large jar with lid	

2:00 pm Do not eat or drink after 2 o'clock. If you break this rule you could feel quite ill later.

Get your Epsom salts ready. Mix 4 tablespoons in 3 cups water and pour this into a jar. This makes four servings, ¾ cup each. Set the jar in the refrigerator to get ice cold (this is for convenience and taste only).

6:00 pm Drink one serving (¾ cup) of the ice cold Epsom salts. If you did not prepare this ahead of time, mix 1 tablespoon in ¾ cup water now. You may add ⅛ teaspoon vitamin C powder to improve the taste. You may also drink a few mouthfuls of water afterwards or rinse your mouth.

Get the olive oil and grapefruit out to warm up.

8:00 pm Repeat by drinking another ¾ cup of Epsom salts. You haven't eaten since two o'clock, but you won't feel hungry. Get your bedtime chores done. The timing is critical for success; don't be more than 10 minutes early or late.

9:45 pm Pour ½ cup (measured) olive oil into the pint jar. Squeeze the grapefruit by hand into the measuring cup. Remove pulp with fork. You should have at least ½ cup, more (up to ¾ cup) is best. You may top it up with fizzy lemonade. Add this to the olive oil. Close the jar tightly with the lid and shake hard until watery (only fresh grapefruit juice does this).

Now visit the bathroom one or more times, even if it makes you late for your ten o'clock drink. Don't be more than 15 minutes late.

10:00 pm Drink the olive oil mixture you have mixed. Take four Ornithine capsules (optional) with the first sips to make sure you will sleep through the night. Take eight if you already suffer from insomnia. Drinking through a large plastic straw helps it go down easier. You may use ketchup, cinnamon, or brown sugar to chase it down between sips. Take it to your bedside if you want, but drink it standing up. Get it down within five minutes (fifteen minutes for very elderly or weak persons).

Lie down immediately. You might fail to get stones out if you don't. The sooner you lie down the more stones you will get out. Be ready for bed ahead of time. Don't clean up the kitchen. As soon as the drink is down walk to your bed and lie down flat for at least 20 minutes. You may feel a train of stones travelling along the bile ducts like marbles. There is no pain because the bile duct valves are open (thank you Epsom salts!). Go to sleep: you may fail to get stones out if you don't.

Next morning. Upon awakening take your third dose of Epsom salts. If you have indigestion or nausea wait until it is gone before drinking the Epsom salts. You may go back to bed. Don't take this potion before 6:00am.

Two Hours Later. Take your fourth (the last) dose of Epsom salts. Drink ¾ cup of this mixture. You may go back to bed.

After Two More Hours you may eat. Start with fruit juice. Half an hour later eat fruit. One hour later you may eat regular food but keep it light. By supper you should feel recovered.

How well did you do?
Expect diarrhea in the morning. Use a flashlight to look for gallstones in the toilet with the bowel movement. Look for the green kind since this is proof that they are genuine gallstones, not food residue. Only bile from the liver is pea green. The bowel movement sinks but gallstones float because of the cholesterol inside. Count them all roughly whether tan or green. You will need to total 2000 stones before the liver is clean enough to rid you of allergies or bursitis or upper back pains permanently. The first cleanse may rid you of them for a few days, but as the stones

from the rear travel forward, they give you the same symptoms again. You may repeat cleanses at two week intervals. Never cleanse when you are ill.

Sometimes the bile ducts are full of cholesterol crystals that did not form into round stones. They appear as a 'chaff' floating on top of the toilet bowl water. It may be tan coloured, harbouring millions of tiny white crystals. Cleansing this chaff is just as important as purging stones.

Once you have finished this programme, I would strongly advise taking Acidophilus, the good bacteria in the gut which helps with good digestion. These good bacteria are found in natural live yoghurt but you will need a more concentrated supplement from the health shop for 2-4 weeks, to replace those cleaned out by the Epsom Salts.   Judy

CONGRATULATIONS

You have taken out your gallstones **without surgery!** I like to think I have perfected this recipe, but I certainly can not take credit for its origin. It was invented hundreds, if not thousands of years ago.

THANK YOU, HERBALISTS!
"Dr Hulda Clark"

Taken from Dr Hulda Clark's-"Cure for all diseases"

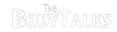

CHAPTER 12

IF YOU CANNOT LOSE WEIGHT
THE TWO MENACES

LOW THYROID FUNCTION AND CANDIDA ALBICANS

If you have found it impossible to lose weight over the years despite repeated diets and vigorous exercise, you might be suffering from one of the following disorders. Often people with these conditions have always been very careful healthy eaters. Yet they can never lose weight and are possibly continuing to put it on, despite eating very little.

These two common disorders are an unrecognised low thyroid function or an over growth of the yeast organism that lives within all of us called Candida Albicans. Both must be treated before you can lose weight or absolutely nothing you do in the way of dieting or exercise will make one jot of difference.

LOW THYROID FUNCTION

Both conditions will give you similar symptoms but there are subtle differences. Both will make you feel very tired and lethargic. Even going for a walk can come to feel like a huge effort. Both cause you to blow up and retain huge amounts of fluid. However, the treatment of the two conditions is very different and it is important to identify which of them you may be suffering with, if at all. The following questionnaire will help you discover if you have one of these two conditions. A low thyroid can give you any of the following symptoms. You may not have them all but if you have several that are severe, you should definitely get further treatment and request a thyroid test from your doctor. An excellent book to help you treat this disorder is called 'The Diet Cure', by Julia Ross. She lists some common symptoms and risk factors of low thyroid function as:

Common symptoms of low thyroid function
- Uncomfortably heavy since childhood
- Family history of thyroid problems
- As a child, played quietly rather than physically
- Weight gain began when you got your period or gave birth, began menopause or after a starvation diet
- Low energy, fatigue, lethargy, need lots of sleep, trouble getting going in the morning
- Tendency to feel cold, particularly in hands and feet
- Tendency to excessive weight gain or inability to lose weight
- Hoarseness, gravely voice
- Depression
- Low blood pressure
- Menstrual problems
- Poor concentration and memory
- Swollen eyelids and face, general water retention
- Thinning or loss of outside of eyebrows
- Tend to have a low temperature
- Headaches (including migraines)
- High cholesterol
- Lump in throat, trouble swallowing (e.g. pills)
- Slow body movement or speech

The medical blood tests for thyroid are fallible and notoriously unreliable. Some of the difficulty with the medical test for Thyroid Stimulating Hormone (TSH) is that the accepted medical range for normal is so wide that a person can drop up to 30% off their normal and still be within this range. The actual level in your body changes at any given time according to how much your body needs at that time. Because this range is considered to be medically acceptable, your doctor will tell you that the level is not bad enough to need attention, despite how you might be feeling. Even a drop of 10% in thyroid levels can result in symptoms such as weight gain, fatigue or hair loss, but this cannot be detected unless a healthy base level has previously been established! Perhaps we should all have thyroid tests done while we are healthy so we have something to measure it against should we ever need to!

CANDIDA ALBICANS

Candida or candidiasis is a condition that occurs when your body loses control of yeast moulds, which exist in all of our digestive tracts. The most common of these yeasts is called candida albicans, although many other microbes including parasites and amoeba may also be involved. These yeasts, even when kept in control in our systems by a healthy immune system and good beneficial bacteria in our guts such as acidophilus and bifidus, are never beneficial. They are parasitic. In a healthy body they are harmless. Candida lives on any mucosal surface of the throat and nose, the vagina and in the gut. If for some reason your immune system is compromised or you are subjected to a strong or repetitive course of antibiotics, which kills off the good bacteria, the candida can flourish out of control. Candida feeds off undigested sugars and starch and changes from yeast to a fungus. The fungus produces toxins, gases and waste products and sometimes alcohol. The adult form of this fungus develops hyphae or long filaments and roots, which are able to penetrate through the mucosal lining of the gut and cause what is called 'leaky gut syndrome'. This allows the toxins to enter the blood stream along with undigested food molecules, causing the body to react with an autoimmune response. The resulting inflammation, bloating and excess mucous production combined with the effects of the toxins on the brain and central nervous system, lead to many symptoms of unwellness and overweight. The most common symptoms of these are:

- Unexplained fatigue
- Weight gain, bloating and fluid retention
- Flatulence and abdominal bloating
- Food cravings, particularly for bread and sugar
- Recurrent thrush or cystitis
- Rectal itching
- Constipation
- Poor memory, lack of concentration, spaced out feelings and mood swings
- Depression and irritability
- Fungal infections on skin or under nails

Many of these symptoms are similar or identical to those caused by low thyroid function and only a skilled practitioner will be able to tell the difference. Cold hands and feet will usually accompany a low thyroid function, which is not present with candida. In both cases you will need to find a health professional to help you. You will usually get short shift from conventional medicine with regard to candida. The condition cannot be neatly defined and is easily confused with other disorders related to the digestion and hormonal imbalances. It is difficult to prove scientifically as yeasts exist naturally in our bodies. Symptoms are wide ranging and often found throughout the body making it difficult to connect them to a single cause. Although the alternative and complimentary medicine field has now been successfully treating candida for 40 years, with thousands of case histories proving its existence and specific mode of treatment, medical tests for candida have only recently become available. Most doctors still refuse to accept its existence. The secondary impact of the toxins and leaky gut syndrome require a prolonged disciplined approach to bring about a complete recovery, something that the drug driven conventional medical world is not set up to pursue. Both these conditions require in-depth and specific treatment, which warrant a book of their own, and many books have indeed already been written on them.

I recommend two excellent books if you would like to investigate these conditions further. The best book to get for natural treatment and information on medical intervention for the thyroid is called 'The Diet Cure' by Julia Ross. There are many good books on Candida, probably the most simple and effective programme is found in 'Beating Candida with Diet' by Gill Jacobs. My tried and tested Candida programme is included here, if you suspect you have it. It is similar to Stage One of the Body Talks but a little stricter in eliminating all sugars, starches and fruit.

I have treated both these conditions successfully in many clients but they are not as common as many people would wish! In many cases, clients were just suffering from bad eating habits, stress, a terrible lifestyle and a lack of knowledge and discipline about healthy eating and food. The statistical occurrence of candida in my clinic over three years has been only about 80 cases in 2000 clients. The low thyroid function condition is even lower at around 40 cases. Before you panic and rush to your doctor, follow the Body Talks Candida programme for two months and then assess your success. Candida is best pursued with the help of a nutritionist, kinesiologist or naturopath.

Although thyroid function should first be investigated medically, complimentary medicine can be very effective in supporting allopathic medicine in treating this disorder.

The Candida Albicans/Yeast Control Programme

There must be a four-stage approach to bring about long term healing.

- Kill off Candida Albicans and significantly reduce the yeast population of the body with supplements and/or pharmaceuticals.
- Starve the yeasts and Candida by eating fewer carbohydrates, starches and sugars and raising the intake of protein and fat.
- Strengthen the immune system.
- Rebuild the health of the intestinal tract, which may have been damaged by an extensive yeast and/or parasite infection.

It is impossible to overcome yeasts without eliminating certain foods which promote its growth and proliferation in the body. It is also vital to eat the good foods with potent anti-yeast qualities. The good news is that the allowed diet does have variety and that this diet does not go on for ever.

Foods you can eat! (Unless intolerant to them)
Meat
Fish
Shellfish
Poultry (organic or freerange variety with low antibiotic content only)
Eggs
Goat's cheese, unsweetened live cow's milk yoghurt, butter
Pulses, beans, lentils, (one medium serving per day only)
Vegetables (except potatoes, yams and tomatoes)
2 small apples a day
3 or 4 Ryvita a day

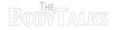

Good Anti-yeast, Anti-fungal foods
Avocado
Broccoli
Brussels sprouts
Cabbage
Cinnamon, cloves, oregano, rosemary, sage, thyme, turmeric
Coconut milk
Fresh lemon juice
Garlic
Extra virgin olive oil
Onions

FOODS TO AVOID
Alcohol and yeast-containing foods: alcohol, baker's and brewer's yeast.
Dairy: Milk and cheese from cows, cottage cheese, sweetened yoghurt.
Fermented food products: all vinegars, hops, malt, soya sauce, pickles, condiments.
Fruit: Just in the beginning you won't be able to eat any fresh fruit at all, other than your daily allowance of 2 small apples, let alone dried fruit or fruit juices (which are also worth avoiding in the long term).
Processed meats: all processed and smoked meats, bacon, sausages, corned beef, ham, MSG and others. This is good long-term advice-full of preservatives and fat.
Starches: all grains including bread, biscuits, gravies, muffins, pancakes, pasta, sauces, waffles and chips. After the first few months you will be able to have a little whole brown rice and millet. It is important to do this diet strictly so it is effective for three months, in order to be able to reintroduce some moderate starch again into your diet as soon as possible.
Sweets and sugar: chocolate, confectionary, fizzy and carbonated drinks, diet drinks, sugar, honey, sweeteners, ketchup.
Potatoes, rice, tomatoes, popcorn
Tea and coffee

Try and be as strict as possible but if you slip, don't despair: just stay on the programme, you haven't blown it. The supplements will still be working.

Other steps:
- Drink eight glasses of water a day. Squeeze a little lemon juice into the water and drink it before meals to support the liver in its yeast-expulsion effort. Other liquids to enjoy are vegetable juices and herbal teas (ginger, mint or Rooibos).
- Use herbs and spices for flavour and marinate in live yoghurt.
- Make up a salad dressing using virgin olive oil and fresh lemon juice.
- Eat as much fresh garlic as possible

Recommended Supplements
- 20 days Aloe Ferox bitter crystals (a powerful anti-fungal agent)
- Multiflora containing lactobacillus-bifidus and acidophilus. Take maximum as directed on label on an empty stomach before meals.
- Pau d'arco. This South American herb contains three anti-yeast and candida compounds.
- Biotin is a B-vitamin that helps stop sugar cravings and has a good inhibitory effect on yeasts- 1000mcg per day
- L-Glutamine 500mg x 4 capsules a day. Take on empty stomach with water between meals, 2 on rising, 2 mid afternoon around 3.30pm
- Lecithin granules or capsules 1200mg daily

The Candida Diet
1. Eat in above ratio every 3 to 4 hours, ie. 3 meals and 2 snacks a day
2. Always eat breakfast. You have gone 10-12 hours overnight without protein.
3. Eat a minimum of 1700 (female) and 2000 (male) calories a day if you want to lose weight. Eat 2100 (female) or 2400 (male) to maintain a healthy stable weight. Eat LOTS of the things you can eat and do not go hungry. After about 3 to 4 weeks you may have days of wanting to eat very little. This is OK: your body is detoxing and needs a rest. Do not force yourself to eat at this stage if you really don't want it.
4. Eat plenty of good fats in your diet including virgin olive oil, nuts and seeds, fish (salmon 3-4 times a week slows down ageing and is very good for you), avocado, butter and eggs.

You will need to follow this programme strictly for 4-6 months. Then adopt stage 2 of the body talks until you reach your ideal weight.

Case History: Overweight, Fatigue, Bloated
Female, Age 53, Blood group O

Following an operation for breast cancer, I was as you can imagine feeling pretty low and a little depressed. My whole body was constantly tired, bloated, overweight and in need of help.

Time and time again when meeting friends, the name Judy Cole came up in conversation. She was a 'lifesaver, someone who could change your life', I was told. Of course I was sceptical. Nevertheless, intrigued, I called to make an appointment.

On hearing Judy tell me that she would 'just talk to my body', during that first appointment, my instinct was to laugh out loud! What did this woman take me for, an idiot? How did she manage to dupe so many intelligent people I thought... but boy was I wrong! Judy Cole has changed my life! Within a month of following the programme strictly I noticed startling improvements. I went through several periods of detox and now here I am four years later, looking and feeling on top of the world. No more bloating, no more swollen joints, no longer feeling tired and listless, no longer looking in the mirror and seeing dried and sallow skin, but above all else she has given me a new sense of energy and well being.

Case History: Candida
Anna, age 13, Blood group B

Anna weighed 98kg when she first came to see me in October 2001. She had always been an overweight child and her body confirmed that she had had a Candida overgrowth for seven years. Anna followed the candida control programme strictly for three months, quite an achievement for a girl of just 13. Two months later the Candida had gone and Anna had lost an astounding 12.5kg! She adopted the Stage One Body Talks programme for a further two months and then stage two. By July 2002 she had lost 30kgs in total. She quickly blossomed as her confidence, self-esteem and sense of well being reached a new level.

I have seen around 11 children with candida and have treated several adults who have battled obesity all their lives due to this insidious condition which had never been detected or correctly treated.

Case History: Candida
Mark, age 57

One such case was a man of 57 who consulted me in Dubai in June 2002 from the UK. Mark had been clinically obese from the age of 11. Despite repeated dieting for many years, which involved mainly low fat, low carbohydrate diets and high exercise programmes he had never had any significant weight loss and had put the lost weight back on very quickly. He recently suffered a cardiac arrest due to his weight and had been diagnosed with late onset Diabetes II. He said he had felt tired all his life though despite this had become a very successful inventor and business man.

His body confirmed that he had suffered a severe candida overgrowth for 47 years and his colon function, which the body indicated to me was only 60%, indicated a sluggish bowel movement and a low good bacteria level of multiflora. But most surprisingly his pancreas registered full normal function and on closer questioning his body told me that the high sugar level in his blood was not diabetes. The candida was producing huge amounts of its waste product which is a type of alcoholic aldehyde and is itself a super sugar. The insulin, which was being produced normally by the pancreas was not able to convert this toxin but during test for diabetes, it kept showing up as a high sugar level.

By following a strict candida diet and avoiding all sugars for 4 months and then adopting the Body Talks stages, Mark eventually lost a total of 42kgs over a year and most satisfyingly, has never shown signs of gaining it back. His 'diabetes' has gone and his heart function, which originally registered at just 67% when I first treated him due to the heart attack, recovered full function in just over 8 months.

Meal Examples for Candida Diet

Breakfast: Live plain yoghurt with 1 grated apple
- **Plus/Either**: 2 eggs + 1-2 Ryvita (+butter/Olivio spread).
- or: 1-2 eggs + (bacon/turkey bacon) + mushrooms + 1-2 Ryvita.
- or: 2 egg omelette + goat's cheese or mozzarella/ham + mushrooms/onions/peppers/spinach + 1-2 Ryvitas.
- or: 2 Ryvita piled with ham/turkey/beef/chicken/tuna/smoked salmon
- or: 1 smoked mackerel + 1-2 Ryvita

Snacks: 6-8 almonds
One or more of:
- Plain live yoghurt + grated apple
- Ryvita + cold meat/tuna/egg/hummus/smoked salmon
- 1 fruit + 2oz cold meat
- veggie sticks + hummus

Lunch and Dinner:
- Women: 4-5oz protein (1oz = 24grams)
- Men: 5-6oz protein

- e.g. or mix and match: average size serving of poultry, fish, meat or 3 eggs
- e.g.: 2oz goats cheese + 2-4 oz meat/fish/chicken.
- Plus: Unlimited vegetables grown above the ground and/or salad
  Use 15gram portions of root vegetables ie, carrots, squash
  (avoid all starches including potato, rice, corn, until candida is dead)
  Use plenty of olive oil and lemon juice dressing

Include 1/3 -1/2 avocado 3-4 times a week

Pulses, beans, nuts and seeds already contain a mix of protein and carbohydrate and can be added to any meal without altering the balance of the rest of your meal.

Eg
- Chicken, Caesar salad/chef's salad with 1-2 Ryvita (optional)
- 2 Ryvitas + tuna mayonnaise and salad
- salmon or chicken and salad/vegetables
- steak and salad/vegetables etc
- roasts/stir fries/grills/stews (thicken with a little corn or rice flour)

Use plenty of garlic, ginger, herbs, yoghurt, seasoning

Please note: Avoid all diet and low sugar foods which will contain aspartame, very poisonous! Avoid smoked meats. Buy organic or free range meats and chicken.
Farmed salmon is very high in antibiotics and growth hormones. Pay more and get wild salmon. Avoid all processed refined margarines and oils, use **ONLY** butter, olive oil spread and virgin olive oil.

TIPS:
Eat plenty and often, do not go hungry. You need to heal your condition, not starve your body! Be patient with your body and the programme. This programme is the basis of good eating for life long term, learning to eat regularly and in balance and to get used to filling up on good things and not being carbohydrate dependent. After three months, when you should be clear of Candida, you may begin to eat a little brown rice at lunch or dinner and vary your fruit intake according to your intolerances. If you have a lot of weight still to lose, adopt Stage Two of the main programme. If you are happy with your weight loss and are feeling great, you may go onto the Stage Three maintenance programme but beware that Candida is notoriously difficult to completely eliminate and you need to be on constant alert for any return of your old symptoms.

CHAPTER 13

RECIPES

Note: There are some recipes that require olive oil. Where posible only use butter for frying.

CREAM OF MUSHROOM SOUP
All blood types
Protein

Ingredients
- ½ large onion, very thinly sliced
- 2 tbsp butter
- 225g button mushrooms, thinly sliced
- juice of one lemon
- 1 tbsp corn flour or potato flour
- 600ml/1 pint chicken stock
- 300ml/½ pint milk
- 150ml dry white wine (optional but will disappear with cooking) or extra stock
- 100ml/4 fl oz fresh double cream
- salt and pepper to taste

1. Heat the butter in a pan and cook the onion gently until transparent. Add the mushrooms and lemon juice and cook them for a couple of minutes; do not let them brown.
2. Add the flour, stir for a minute then gradually add the stock, milk and white wine. Bring the mixture to the boil and simmer gently for 15 minutes.
3. Season to taste and just before serving add the cream and adjust the seasoning.

TUNA AND CHICK-PEA SALAD
All blood types
Protein

Serves 4
This is ideal for unexpected guests because most of the ingredients come from the store-cupboard. Prawns can be used instead of the tuna.

Ingredients
1 x 400g/14oz can chick-peas/garbanzo beans, well rinsed
425g/15oz cooked peas, fresh or frozen
(try 1 apple or mango for a sweeter flavour)
400g/14oz cooked fresh tuna or canned in brine
2 tbsp each of coarsely chopped fresh basil, chives and parsley
juice of ½ lemon
black pepper to taste
2 tbsp olive oil

Mix all the ingredients in bowl and serve at room temperature-or chill if preferred. Excellent served with a salad made with Chinese cabbage and baby spinach leaves.

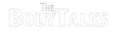

GARLIC CHICKEN (Great for Candida)
Not for B blood types
Protein

Ingredients
- 2 x medium chickens cut into pieces
- 1 large onion, diced
- 2 large carrots, sliced
- 4 sticks of celery, sliced
- 3oz/75g butter
- 20-30 garlic cloves, unpeeled and left whole
- juice of 2 lemons
- pepper to taste

1. Heat the butter in a frying pan and add the onions, carrots and celery. Cook till soft, stirring continuously. Transfer the vegetables to a casserole dish with a tight-fitting lid.
2. Lay the chicken pieces on top and sprinkle with lemon juice and pepper. Put the garlic around and on the chicken. Cover the pot tightly-this is essential, as the chicken must cook in its own juices. Cook in a preheated 180°C/350°F/Gas 4 oven for 1 hour. Do not uncover till ready to serve.

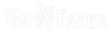

LEMON TARRAGON CHICKEN WITH BUTTON MUSHROOMS
Not for B blood types
Protein

Serves 6
This is one of the most delicious ways to serve chicken. This dish should have a very fragrant smell from the tarragon and the sauce should be well flavoured with the lemon.

Ingredients
- 1 chicken
- 1 large, onion, finely chopped
- butter
- 100g/4oz button mushrooms
- 4 tbsp spelt flour
- chicken stock made during the cooking process
- juice of at least 2 lemons
- Tarragon and black pepper

1. Preheat the oven to 180°C/350°F/Gas 4.
2. Place the chicken in a covered casserole with 1.2 litres water. Poach in the moderate oven for an hour or until the juices run clear when a skewer is jabbed into the thickest part of the thigh. Set aside to cool, reserving the stock for the sauce. This part can be prepared ahead of time and the sauce can be made at the last minute with the chicken chunks swiftly heated through.
3. Cook the onion in the butter in a heavy-bottomed casserole until it is clear and soft, but not coloured. Throw in the button mushrooms, sprinkle with the flour and mix. Remove from the heat and add the stock, lemon juice, plenty of freshly ground black pepper and the tarragon. Place back on a moderate heat and bring to the boil, stirring constantly until thickened. The sauce will take on a slightly greenish colour from the fresh tarragon.
4. Skin the chicken and remove the cooked meat from the bones. Cut the chicken into large chunks and put into the sauce. Heat through over a gentle heat, stirring.
5. Serve with a variety of vegetables and/or a green salad.

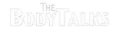

ROAST TURKEY THIGH WITH HONEY AND GINGER GLAZE
All blood types
Protein

It is well worth marinating the turkey for 24 hours before cooking. Not only does the marinade permeate the meat, but it also tenderises it. Leave the bone in the meat. This holds the thigh together during cooking and also adds flavour. The bone can be removed with a sharp knife before carving if you wish. The gravy made from the marinade and cooking juices is delicious.

Ingredients
900g/2lb turkey thigh, with the bone still in
2 tsp corn flour mixed with 1 tbsp water

For the Marinade:
½ tbsp Dijon mustard
½ tbsp tamari soy sauce
1 tbsp orange juice (This little bit will do no harm to your detox programme)
1 tsp ground ginger
1 tbsp runny honey
¾ tbsp olive oil
2 cloves garlic, crushed

1. Mix all the marinade ingredients in a non-metallic bowl. Brush over both sides of the meat and leave for at least 2 hours, maximum 24 hours, before cooking. Cover and store in the refrigerator. Preheat the oven to 180°C/350°F/Gas 4. Put the meat in a roasting pan skin side down. Pour over any remaining marinade and put enough water in the roasting pan to cover the bottom by 6mm/¼in.
2. Allow 40 minutes' cooking time per 450g of turkey. Turn the turkey halfway through cooking and add a little more water to keep the bottom of the pan covered. When the cooking time has been completed, remove from the oven, place the meat on a serving dish and stand for 15 minutes before carving.

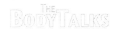

3. Meanwhile, take the roasting pan and add enough liquid (stock or the water used for cooking the vegetables to accompany this meal) to make up to 300ml, ½ pint/or 1 ¼ cups of liquid. Scrape the residue and juices up from the pan and bring to the boil. Strain the gravy into a small saucepan, then return to the heat and adjust seasoning if necessary. Remove from the heat and stir in the corn flour mixture to thicken the gravy.
4. Serve with vegetable and/or green salad.

LEG OF LAMB WITH BEANS AND GREEN PEPPERCORNS
Not for A blood types
Protein

Serves 8
Ingredients
10 large cloves of garlic, peeled but left whole
2 kg lean leg of lamb
2 tbsp butter
400g/14oz fresh spinach
400g/14oz tinned flageolet beans, drained
400g/14oz tinned cannelloni beans, drained
2 sprigs fresh rosemary or 2 tsp dried
handful of green peppercorns

1. Insert 6 garlic cloves into the lamb and put the rest into a heavy casserole dish (one that you can use on the hob) with the butter and the spinach. Cook briskly for 5 minutes. Add the beans, rosemary and peppercorns.
2. Lay the leg of lamb on top of the mixture and cover tightly. The dish can then be cooked very slowly either on the hob or in the oven 150°C/300°F/Gas 2 for 3-4 hours
3. To serve, move lamb onto a serving dish and surround with spinach and bean mixture.

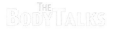

RACK OF LAMB WITH MUSTARD CRUST
Not for A blood types
Protein

Serves 6
This mustard crust gives great flavour to the lamb.

Ingredients
Rack of lamb with at least 12 cutlets, trimmed of most of its fat

For the crust:
25g/1oz melted butter
4 tbsp wholegrain mustard (most mustards have wheat flour in so check the label carefully)
25g/1oz parsley, chopped fine
100g shallots, chopped fine
1 tbsp each of dried rosemary, marjoram, oregano, thyme
3 tbsp dry white wine
1 small pack plain potato crisps

1. Heat oven to 180°C/350°F/Gas 4.
2. Roast the rack of lamb uncovered in a baking tray for 15 minutes for 500g. This will give a slightly pink middle. If you want it more cooked then try 20 minutes per 500g
3. Combine all the crust ingredients except the crisps. Crush the crisps in a bag with a rolling pin.
4. 10 minutes before the meat is ready, take it out and spread the fat side with a thick layer of the mustard mixture. Sprinkle over the crushed crisps and return to the oven for 10 minutes to finish cooking the meat and crisp the crust.

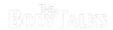

SALMON EN PAPILLOTTE
All blood types
Protein

Serves 6
This dish started life at dinner parties in Victorian India where it could be made with any white fish. If you prefer, substitute fillets of hake or halibut for the salmon. It needs to marinade overnight so start the dish the day before you need it.

Ingredients
- 6 salmon steaks
- 6 tbsp olive oil
- 50g/2oz shallots, finely chopped
- 2 cloves garlic, finely chopped
- large handful of fresh parsley
- 3 tbsp white wine vinegar or lemon juice
- grated peel of 2 limes
- salt and pepper

1. Put the fish in a microwave/heatproof dish, cover with boiling water and simmer for 5 minutes on a hob or 2 minutes in the microwave. Drain carefully and set aside.
2. Mix all the remaining ingredients in a large glass dish (enough to hold the fish comfortably) Lay the fish on top of the marinade and spoon over excess so that the steaks are immersed. Cover and leave for 6-12 hours.
3. To cook the fish, lay the steaks with their marinade in an ample bed of foil and cover them with well-oiled greaseproof paper. The fish can them be cooked on a barbeque, under a hot grill or in a wide heavy frying pan. It should take between 6 and 8 minutes, depending on the thickness of the steaks.

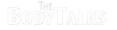

TUNA CURRY WITH CORIANDER AND COCONUT

(This contains intolerances for all blood types in small doses but would be fine as an occasional cheat once over initial detox. Any other meat or fish can be substituted).

Protein

Serves 6

Ingredients
- 3 tins of tuna in olive oil or brine
- 2 leeks, trimmed and sliced thinly
- 2cm root ginger, peeled and sliced
- 5 large cloves garlic, peeled and thinly sliced
- 1 small green chilli, deseeded and sliced (optional)
- 2 green peppers deseeded and sliced
- 3 tbsp mild curry powder
- 400g/14oz tin of chick peas, drained
- 400g/14oz tin of coconut milk
- 2 handfuls coriander leaves, chopped
- juice of 2-3 limes or lemons

1. Drain the oil or brine from the tuna. Add the tuna to a heavy wide pan. Add the leeks, ginger root, garlic, chilli, green pepper and curry powder and fry together for 3-4 minutes.
2. Add the chickpeas and coconut milk, bring to the boil and simmer covered for 10 minutes. Add the tuna fish and cook for a further 5 minutes.
3. Finally add the lemon or lime juice to taste and season if required.
4. Serve the curry liberally sprinkled with the fresh coriander leaves and a green salad. Rice can be served in stage 2 and 3.

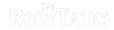

ROMAN CABBAGE
All Blood types
Good carbohydrates with a little protein from the pine nuts.

Serves 4
Ingredients
- 100g brown rice
- 15g/½oz butter
- 1 onion finely sliced
- 450g/1lb Savoy cabbage, chopped
- 150ml/¼pint water or vegetable stock
- 50g/2oz pine nuts
- 10 coriander seeds or chopped fresh coriander
- 25g/1oz butter
- salt and pepper

1. Cook the rice according to packet instructions.
2. Cook the onion gently in the butter. Add cabbage and mix well before adding the stock or water and a little seasoning. Cover and simmer for 15 minutes.
3. Turn the cabbage into an oven-proof dish. Stir the pine nuts and coriander seeds into the rice and season if required. Spread the mixture over the cabbage in the dish and dot the top with butter. Cover and cook in a moderate oven (180°C/350°F/Gas 4) for 20 minutes to allow flavours to amalgamate before serving.

WILD MUSHROOMS AND AUTUMN VEGETABLES (WITH POTATO CAKES)
All blood types
Good carbohydrates

This is a very rich dish and is ideal for festive occasions. The potato cakes are optional in stages 2 and 3 only. Button or chestnut mushrooms will do just as well. The recipe calls for oil so it doesn't burn but butter can still be substituted. The secret is to prepare all the vegetables ahead of time and cook them just before serving. The vegetables should be only just cooked and still have a certain 'bite'; they will go mushy if they are overcooked.

Ingredients

FOR THE AUTUMN VEGETABLES:
- 170g carrots
- 275g artichokes
- 2 tbsp olive oil
- ½ tbsp balsamic vinegar

FOR THE MUSHROOMS:
- 100g/4oz shiitake mushrooms, sliced
- 100g/4oz field mushrooms, quartered
- 100g/4oz wild mushrooms of your choice, left whole
- 2 level tablespoons of butter
- 115g/1½oz spring onions/scallions cut into 2.5m/1 in pieces
- good pinch cayenne pepper
- 1½ tbsp lemon juice
- freshly ground black pepper to taste
- 2 cloves garlic, finely sliced
- 1½ tbsp tomato puree/paste (optional)
- a big handful flat parsley with stalks, chopped

FOR THE POTATO CAKES:
450g/1 lb potatoes
1 egg beaten
1/8 tsp freshly grated nutmeg
plenty of black pepper to taste
30g/1oz fine oatmeal to dust
butter for frying

1. Preheat the oven to its highest setting. Peel and slice the vegetables. Slice the carrots diagonally to half the thickness of the artichokes. I would suggest that the carrots be sliced 3 mm 1/8 in thick and the artichokes 6mm/1/4 in thick. Put the slices into a mixing bowl and pour over the oil and vinegar. Toss so that the vegetables are coated then spread out in a roasting tray so that there is only one layer of vegetables. Roast for 20 minutes. When cooked the vegetables should not be soft, but still have a bit of bite.
2. Meanwhile, prepare the potatoes. Boil them until they are soft. Drain, peel and mash off the heat. Stir in the beaten egg and the seasoning. Divide the mixture into 4 portions. With your hands, form flat patties. Put the oatmeal on to a plate and carefully coat the flat surfaces of the potato cakes.
3. While the potatoes are boiling and the carrots and artichokes are roasting, prepare the mushroom ingredients.
4. When the carrots and artichokes are ready and the potato cakes have been formed, get 2 frying pans and assemble the dish. This will only take about 5 minutes.
5. In one frying pan heat just enough sunflower oil to coat the bottom of the pan and fry the potato cakes in the medium hot oil, turning when golden and crispy.
6. In the other frying pan heat the butter for the mushrooms. Put in the spring onions and stir-fry for 1 minute. Add the cayenne pepper, the lemon juice, black pepper and garlic and cook, stirring for another minute. Add the tomato puree (optional) and stir to mix well. Add the mushrooms, cooked carrots and artichokes and fry, turning the ingredients over constantly for a couple of minutes or until cooked through but still firm. Stir in the roughly chopped parsley, adjust seasoning to taste and serve immediately with meat, chicken or fish. In stage 2 or 3, also serve with the hot potato cake or brown rice.

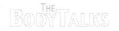

SLOW ROAST VEGETABLES WITH HALLOUMI CHEESE
All blood types
Good carbohydrates with protein. A perfectly balanced dish.

This dish is so delicious and so healthy, make it a regular favourite.

Serves 4
Ingredients
- 50g/2oz butter
- Selection of vegetables from mushrooms, peppers, courgettes, broccoli, cauliflower, beans, butternut squash, carrots, etc
- Juice of 1 lemon
- Salt and black pepper
- Fresh rosemary
- 2 tablespoons virgin olive oil
- Packet of Halloumi cheese

1. Preheat oven to 180C/350F/Gas 4.
2. Chop all vegetables into bite size chunks and place in large baking tin. Sprinkle with little chunks of butter, lemon juice and rosemary to taste. Season with salt and pepper.
3. Cover with foil and roast in oven for 20 minutes.
4. Add 1 inch chunks of Halloumi cheese, remove foil cover and return to oven for a further 20 minutes. Shake tin from time to time to prevent sticking to the bottom of the pan.

Serve alone or with a green salad

CHOCOLATE CAKE WITH MINNEOLAS-SAUCE
All blood types
Starch and sugar

(sauce can also be done with grapefruits or pommelos)

Ingredients
200g/7oz dark chocolate 74% of cacao (melt in waterbath (bain-marie)
50g/2oz unsalted butter
8 eggs separated
5tbsp fine brown sugar

Add egg-yolks to the sugar and beat until light yellow. Mix the melted chocolate and the melted butter with the beaten egg-yolks and sugar, beat egg-white and add successively.

Place the cake in a waterbath in the oven. Bake in middle of oven at 170°C/325°F/Gas 3 in the middle for 30 to 40 minutes.

Mineolas-sauce

8 mineolas
1 tbsp peel from mineolas
5 tbsp of brown sugar
1 tbsp of icing sugar
1 tbsp of unsalted butter

Peel the mineolas, cut in slices without the white skin, keep juice. Cut peel of mineolas into small slices. Melt the butter in a small pan, add sugar, peels and juice. After the liquid gets thicker add slices of mineolas. Cook for approx. 10-15 minutes until the sauce is still a little liquid-stir gently with a wooden spoon.

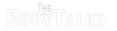

HOT CHOCOLATE SOUFFLÉ (Stages 2 and 3 only!)
All blood types
All sugar, eat in small portions!

Serves 4

Although this is light it is seriously rich.

Ingredients:
    5 egg whites
    small pinch salt
    200g castor sugar
    50g cocoa powder
    few drops vanilla essence
    double cream or Greek yoghurt to serve with soufflé

1. Heat the oven to 180°C/350°F/Gas 4 and put in a Bain Marie big enough to hold the soufflé dish. Allow the water to get warm as you heat the oven. Lightly grease the soufflé dish
2. Whisk the egg whites with the salt until pretty stiff. Whisk 3 tablespoons of the sugar then fold in the rest with the cocoa powder and the vanilla.
3. Spoon the mixture into the soufflé dish and cook in the Bain Marie for 30-40 minutes until it is risen and crisp on top
4. Serve at once with cream or Greek yoghurt

FUDGY NUT CAKE (Stage 3 only)
All blood types
High sugar

This is unbelievably delicious and flourless, fattening, should be eaten with respect in small portions.

Ingredients:
- 350g plain chocolate, chopped
- 175g unsalted butter, diced
- 55g cocoa powder
- 5 large eggs
- 1 tsp real vanilla essence
- 250g golden caster sugar
- 100g mixture of nuts, roughly chopped
- icing sugar and cocoa for dusting

One 22cm spring-form pan, greased and base-lined. Set oven to 180°C/350°F/Gas 4.

1. Put the chopped chocolate and diced butter into a heatproof bowl set over a pan of steaming water. Stir frequently until melted and smooth. Remove from the heat, stir in the cocoa, then leave to cool.
2. Meanwhile in a large heat-proof bowl, whisk the eggs, vanilla and sugar briefly until frothy. Set the bowl over a pan of steaming water-the water should not touch the base of the bowl. Using an electric hand whisk, whisk the mixture until it is very pale and thick-when the whisk is lifted it should leave a visible ribbon-like trail.
3. Remove the bowl from the heat, and whisk for a couple minutes so the mixture cools. Using a large metal spoon, carefully fold in the chocolate mixture, followed by the nuts
4. When thoroughly combined, spoon into the prepared spring-form pan and smooth the surface.
5. Bake in the preheated oven for about 35 minutes or until firm to the touch but moist inside (do not overcook or the cake will be dry and hard to slice).
6. Let cool in the tin, turn out and serve, dusted with cocoa and icing sugar. Store in an airtight container and eat within 1 week. It does not freeze well.

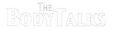

ALMOND COOKIES
All blood types
Starch and sugar

Portion: a maximum of two a day.
Makes 12-15 small cookies

These crumbly little cookies melt in the mouth. They are treats, not to be made or eaten in stage 1 of your programme.

Ingredients
- 90g spelt flour
- 30g ground almonds
- 75g butter
- 30g fructose sugar or 35g of white sugar
- 1 tsp almond extract
- 1 egg, beaten
- 55g flaked almonds

1. Put the flour, ground almonds, butter and fructose into a food processor with the blade attachment and pulse until the mixture resembles crumbs. Add the almond extract and 2 tbsp of the beaten egg. As soon as the dough forms a ball, take it out. Knead slightly. The dough will be soft and slightly sticky. Roll into a ball, wrap and refrigerate for at least 1 hour.
2. Preheat the oven to 160°C/325°F/Gas 3.
3. Flour a surface and a rolling pin and roll the dough out as thinly as possible. Using a pastry brush, lightly coat the surface of the dough with the remaining egg. Sprinkle over the flaked almonds and roll in lightly with the rolling pin. Cut with a cookie cutter and carefully arrange on a baking sheet.
4. Bake for 15 minutes until a light golden brown. Do not allow to darken.
5. Cool on a wire rack.

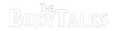

CAPE SEED LOAF
All blood types
Good starch
An easy loaf to make for bread beginners

Ingredients
- 500g spelt flour
- 85g sunflower seeds
- 50g pumpkin seeds
- 25g poppy seeds
- 350ml lukewarm water
- 1 egg beaten
- 1 tsp salt
- 7g yeast (1 easy blend packet)
- 1 tbsp castor sugar
- 2 tbsp olive oil
- poppy & sesame seeds to decorate

1. Mix flour, seed, salt, yeast and sugar in a large bowl. Drizzle olive oil over the mixture and stir in warm water to make a soft dough. Knead in the bowl for one minute
2. Lift dough into an oiled loaf tin (19cm x 9cm). Press in with your knuckles and make a shallow dent down the centre of the loaf (so it rises evenly)
3. Brush the top with egg and sprinkle over alternate lines of poppy and sesame seeds. Cover with a cloth and leave to rise until almost at the top of the tin (20-30) minutes.
4. Preheat the oven to 180C/360F/Gas 4. Bake for 45-50 minutes. Cool on rack

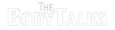

SPELT MUFFINS
All blood types
Starch

Portion: one a day
Ingredients
- 2½ cups Spelt flour
- 1 to 1½ cups milk
- 3 eggs beaten
- ¼ cup sugar or honey
- 1 tbsp baking powder
- 1 tbsp olive oil
- ½ tsp salt if desired

1. Combine all the dry ingredients. Add milk, oil and eggs. Mix well
2. Fill muffin trays and bake in oven 190°C/375°F/Gas 5 for 15 minutes or until browned
3. You could add cinnamon, all spice, ½ cup chopped almonds or hazelnuts if desired

SPELT PIE CRUST
All blood types
Starch

Ingredients
- 1 cup + 2 tbsp Spelt flour
- 3 tbsp olive oil
- 2 tbsp cold water
- ½ tsp salt

1. Whisk oil, water and salt together
2. Stir in the flour and mix until evenly moistened. Press onto a 9" pie plate and bake the empty crust for 12 minutes

SPELT-BREAD RECIPE FOR KENWOOD BREADMAKER

Use the same method, just change the ingredients as follows:

Ingredients	Large	Regular
egg	1 plus 1 egg yolk	1
water	see method	see method
clear honey or sugar	30ml (5 tsp)	15ml (3 tsp)
lemon juice	15ml (3 tsp)	10ml (2 tsp)
spelt flour white	250g	200g
spelt flour dark	250g	175g
skimmed milk powder	5 tsp	3 tsp
salt	2 tsp	1½ tsp
easy blend dried yeast	1½ tsp	1 tsp

Makes 1 large or regular loaf

Follow the method of your Kenwood Bread Machine (whole-wheat Cycle) Programme 4 & 5

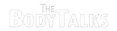

RECOMMENDED READING

"Atkins for Life The Next Level" by R. C. Atkins ISBN 1 405 02110 1

"Beat Candida through Diet" by Gill Jacobs ISBN 0 0918 1545 2

"Eat Right 4 your Type" by Dr. Peter J D'Adamo ISBN 0 3991 4255 X

"Enter the Zone" Barry Sears ISBN 0 06039150 2

"Love, Medicine and Miracles" by Bernie Siegel ISBN 0 0996 3270 5

"Loving What is" by Byron Katie ISBN

"The Diet Cure" by Julia Ross ISBN 0 7181 4397 3

"Thyroid Power" by Richard L Shames and Karilee Shames ISBN 0 688 17236 9

"Spontaneous Healing" by Andrew Weil MD. ISBN 0 8041 1794 2

"The Schwarzbein Principle" by Diana Schwarzbein, MD. ISBN 1 55874 680 3

CONTACTS

Other book in the series: "The Body Talks", Vital food facts and 90 Day Diet Diary

For more information on Judy Cole's work see: www.judycole.co.uk
Aloe Ferox bitter crystals for the bowel available to order on this website. See page 79.

ACKNOWLEDGMENTS

First and foremost my deepest thanks to all my clients who have faithfully followed this programme. Your bodies showed us the way but your dedication proved it works.

James Whelan, Will Rankin and Ann Gardner for their superb editing.

To all my teachers, who came into my life at the perfect time and taught me exactly what I needed to know to move to the next stage of my development. To Annie Watts, who introduced me to deep tissue massage and gave me the tools to work with professional sport. Kai Chi, for teaching me to feel energy and injury in the body like an xray. To Wayne Morton, the former Yorkshire and England cricket physiotherapist, who allowed me to work with him. Sue Woods, my superb Touch for Health teacher. Guido and Mia Swartz in South Africa, who opened up the world of dowsing to me. You are all masters of your fields and I am so privileged to have been your pupil.

To Ewan Cameron, whose enduring support and love, pushed me to fulfil my potential.

Diane Mineault, for her encouragement, belief and friendship. And to my many other friends through the years, who have been so loyal.

To Dr Ralph Banning, Dr Lee Too, Josie and Militon, my brilliant guides and mentors.

And to my wonderful parents, to whom this book is specially dedicated. You have always been there, no matter how unorthodox my ideas became. Your faith in my gift never wavered, even when mine did!

To all of you, thank you.

Index The Body Talks

A
A blood type, 30, 59
AB blood type, 34
accelerated metabolic aging
    alcohol and, 104
    insulin and, 70
acidophilus, yeast overgrowth and, 154, 157
acne, 23, 37, 147
activity levels and exercise, 16, 20
addictions,
    carbohydrate consumption and, 53, 54
    insulin and, 65
    overcoming, 116
adrenal glands, 22, 82, 83, 85, 109
alcohol
    allowance, 104, 115
    calories, 104
    cholesterol and, 66
    insulin and, 70
    most yeast free, 40
alcoholism, 62
alfalfa, 129
allergies, 23, 39, 136, 147, 150
almonds, 45, 51, 134
almond cookies recipe, 182
Aloe Ferox Crystals, 38, 79
amino acids, 45, 46, 124
    L-glutathione, 129
    L-glutamine, 131
    L-tyrosine, 131
aniseed tea, 143
anorexia, 18
Asian cuisine, restaurants, 120, 122
aspartame, 100, 126, 134
Atkins R C, 186
avocados, 59, 61, 64, 68, 80, 99, 129, 134, 161

B
B blood type, 7, 32, 137
balanced diet, 72, 73, 88
barley, 45, 60, 62, 141
beef, 30, 50
better butter recipe, 43
bifidus, 148, 157, 162

bile
    digestion and, 66, 76, 80
    liver cleanse and, 39, 150
    skimmed milk and, 63
biopsy
    coeliac disease, 141
blood antibodies, 22
blood sugar
    balancing, 74
    diabetes and, 71
hyperglycaemia, 75
    hypoglycaemia and, 75
insulin and, 70
snacks and, 101
    supplements, 131
blood tests
    candida albicans and, 158
coeliac disease and, 141
    food intolerance and, 25
    Nutron test and, 25
thyroid and, 156
Body fat, 18
    alcohol and, 105
    calories and, 81
sugar and, 53, 75, 144
fats and, 61, 138
insulin and, 70, 74
metabolic rate and, 72
bone formation, 44, 46
    loss, 47, 81
bowels,
constipation and, 38, 138
detox and, 38
    diarrhea and, 38
    IBS, 19, 24, 38, 80
brain chemistry, 7
    B12 and, 33, 128, 149
    diets and, 17, 20, 101
    protein and, 76
sugar and, 75, 104
bread, 40, 42, 52, 54, 60, 78
bread machine wheat free bread recipe, 185
    spelt muffins recipe, 184
    spelt pie crust recipe, 184
breakfast
    examples of, 48, 96, 97, 110
    importance of, 46, 72, 75, 94

bulimia, 18
B12 vitamin
    brain chemistry and, 33, 128, 149
breast cancer, 63, 136, 145, 160
burgers, 124
butter, 61, 63, 64, 65, 68, 80, 94, 96, 135

C
caffeine
    diabetes and, 70
tea and coffee and, 135, 142, 146
calcium, 47, 63, 69, 80
calorie, 14, 20, 93
    alcohol and, 104
    almonds and, 134
    grains and, 141
    ideal, 76, 81, 88, 94
    metabolic rate and, 46, 72, 81
    starvation mode and, 81, 82, 93, 109
cancer, 68, 129
    breast, 63, 136, 145, 160
    bowel, 78, 141
    chemicals and, 136
Candida Albicans, 155, 157
    alcohol and, 157, 161
canola oil, 62, 65
cape seed loaf recipe, 183
carbohydrates,
    bread, 40, 42, 52, 54, 60, 78
bad, 60,
    candida albicans and, 157
    cravings and, 13, 61, 62, 90, 101
    fibre, 78
    fruits, 58
    good, 56
    insulin and, 53, 75, 144
    overeating, 55
    starch, 16, 52, 54, 56, 60, 108
    tips for eating, 55
cayenne pepper, 130
cellular aging, 104, 129, 140, 162
cellular detox, 36
cellulite, 6, 83, 104, 128, 130, 141
cereal, breakfast, 53, 145
chamomile tea, 143
cheese,
    A blood type and, 30

B blood type and, 32
O blood type and, 28
AB blood type and, 34
Good, moderate, bad, 50
Chemicals, 35, 39, 136
diet foods and, 139
immune system and, 14, 16, 17
insulin and, 70
cancer and, 136
fast foods and, 124
food additives and, 139
proteins and, 44
chicken
B blood type and, 32
antibiotics and, 137
Chinese cuisine, restaurants, 120
chocolate, 13, 58, 75,
allowance, 109
soul food, 117
chocolate cake with minneolas sauce recipe, 179
chocolate fudge nut cake recipe, 181
chocolate soufflé recipe, 180
cholesterol, 66
alcohol and, 104
ADH Co-A Reductase and, 67
eggs and, 68
insulin and, 75
heart disease and, 66
livers role in, 67
chromium, 131
CoQ10, 129
coeliac disease, 14, 141
coffee, 24, 42, 96, 135
A blood type and, 30
B blood type and, 32
O blood type and, 28
AB blood type and, 34
complex carbohydrates, 16, 52, 54, 95
constipation, 38, 138
cooking with fats, 140
corn oil, 62, 65
cows milk,
A blood type and, 30
B blood type and, 32
O blood type and, 28
AB blood type and, 34
see lactose

cravings and,
candida albicans and, 157, 162
carbohydrates and, 13, 61, 62, 90, 101, 104
supplements for, 20, 131, 132
cream, 138, 142
cream of mushroom soup, 166

D
D'Adamo, Peter J, 23, 24, 137, 186
dandelion coffee, 143
depression,
candida and, 157
cholesterol and, 66
diets and, 82
omega 3 fats and, 61, 62
thyroid and, 156
desserts,
wheat free, 117
detox,
cellular, 36, 22, 93
digestive, 36
food intolerances and, 20, 23
healing crisis and, 37
liver cleanse and, 150
diabetes, 30, 141
alcohol and, 104
processed fats and, 63
supplements to help, 131
wheat and, 147
diarrhea,
IBS and, 19, 24, 38, 80
dieting,
adrenals and, 22, 82, 88, 109
consequences of, 14
ideal weight and, 76, 81, 88, 94
starvation mode and, 81, 82, 93, 109
weight gain and, 14
yo-yo, 14, 84
weight loss graphs and, 84
dining out,
Arabic restaurants, 120
Chinese restaurants, 120
French restaurants, 121,
Indian restaurants, 122
Italian restaurants, 123
general, 118
drinks, 102

alcohol, 104, 115
diet sodas, 126, 134
juices, 42, 58, 102
water, 38, 102, 118
mixers, 105

E
eating disorders, 18
eggs,
body talks about, 47, 72, 139
cholesterol and, 66, 68
endocrine system, 20, 22, 38, 58, 88
Evening Primrose oil, 130
exercise, 85
calories and, 81, 116
ideal programme, 87
immune system and, 22,
over exercise, 85, 90
extra virgin olive oil, 62, 100

F
fast foods, 124
fats,
bile and, 63, 66, 76, 80
cancer and, 63
cooking with, 140
damaged, 62
essential, 62
good, bad, 64
hydrogenated, 62
milk and, 63
saturated, 65
tips on eating, 65
transfatty acids, 62
fats do not make you fat, 61, 70, 75, 81
fats, damaged and memory loss, 62
fat storage system, 53, 74, 75, 81
fennel tea, 143
fibre, 78
ancestors and, 78
bowels and, 38, 138
vegatables and, 52
sources of good, 52, 144, 146
fibroids, 148
fish,
Celtic blood and, 62
omega 3 and, 62

fizzy drinks,
    artificial sweeteners and, 100, 126, 134
    potassium, sodium balance and, 102
flax seed oil, 62
flour,
    bread, 40, 42, 52, 54, 60, 78
    bread mixer recipe, 183
    rye, 42, 53, 54, 62, 78, 135
    spelt, 54, 78, 135, 141, 146
    wheat, 147
Food and Drug Administration (FDA), 145
French cuisine, restaurants, 121
fruit, 58
    detox diets and, 58
    juice, 58
frying, 140

G
gallstones, 150
garlic chicken recipe, 168
genetically engineered foods, 140
ghee, 140
ginger, 95
    candida albicans and, 162
    herbal tea, 143
ginseng, 143
gluten, 141
    allergy, coeliac, 14, 141
intolerance to, 14
tests for, 141
glycogen, 52, 53, 74, 76
goats cheese, milk, 42, 142
goldenseal tea, 143
gravies, 161

H
headaches, 23, 24, 37, 71, 111, 133,
    chemicals and, 136
coffee and, 135
healing, 8
B12 and, 128
detox, 36
diabetes mellitus II, 70
illnesses, food intolerances and, 23, 24
immune system, 20
the healing stage, 93, 108
your weight and, 10, 14, 17

heart disease, 66
herbal teas, 142, 143
herbs, 53, 78, 95
    cayenne pepper, 130
    turmeric, 130
high carbohydrate, low fat diet, 14
HMG Co-A Reductase, 67
honey, 142
hormones, 61
    balance, 20, 44, 109
    cholesterol and, 66, 67
    detox symptoms, 37
    evening primrose oil, 130
hormones in food, 137, 145, 165
how the body talks, 8, 12
hummus, 102, 119, 120, 125
hydrochloric acid, 76, 147
hydrogenated fats, 62, 65, 66
hypoglycaemia, 75
hypothyroidism, 155
    symptoms, 156
    unrecognized, 156
    weight and, 155

I
ice cream, 142
ideal body composition, 54
ideal weight, 76, 81, 88, 94
immune system,
eating and, 14, 16, 17, 139
exercise and, 22
healing of, 20, 22, 38, 58, 88
insulin resistance
    defined, 70
    from smoking and chemicals, 70
    in fat storage, 75
Irritable Bowel Syndrome, 19, 24, 38, 80
Italian cuisine, restaurants, 123

J
Jacobs, Gill, 186
joints
    food intolerances and, 24, 141, 147
    joint aches and pains, 29, 127, 160
junk food, 124
juice, fruit, 58

K
K vitamin,
acidophilus and,
    fibroids and, 148
kinesiology, 7, 8, 24

L
L-Ornithine, 151
lactose, 41, 42, 52
lactose free desserts, 117
lamb, leg of, with beans and peppercorns, 171
lamb, rack of, with mustard crust, 172
legumes, 45, 51
    butter and, 135
    cream and, 138, 142
    yoghurt and, 148
lemon tarragon chicken recipe, 169
lifestyle, changing, 14, 17, 21, 22, 39
    insulin and, 70
    toxins and, 85
liver,
    cholesterol and, 67
    insulin and, 75
liver cleanse, 150
L-Glutamine, 131
L-Glutathione, 129
low fat diets, 14, 84
    dangers, 81, 82, 93, 109
low blood sugar, 75
lunch,
    examples of, 48, 97, 99, 110
low fat diets,
    dangers of, 14

M
magnesium, 29, 80, 130, 134
maintenance programme, 114
man-made products, 60, 63, 135, 140
meat, 35, 45, 47,
fats in, 61, 64, 77, 80
guideline to eating, 97, 98, 100
protein in, 50, 139
menopause, 144
metabolism,
    defined, 44, 115
    exercise and, 88
    foods and, 46, 61, 72, 81,

Mexican cuisine, restaurants, 123
minerals,
    chromium, 131
magnesium, 130
    potassium, 130
    selenium, 129
iron, 129
moods,
    candida albicans, 157
    eating right, 77
    thyroid, 156
multivitamins,
    see alfalfa
muscle mass,
    gaining, 18, 20, 77, 83, 85
    losing, 14, 46, 72, 75, 81, 82
    metabolic rate, 44, 115
muscle injuries,
    food intolerances and, 147
mushrooms, 56, 78, 97, 98, 99
    mushroom soup recipe, 166
    mushrooms and autumn vegetables recipe, 176

N
New England Journal of Medicine, The, 139
nettle tea, 143
non starchy vegetables, 156
nuts and seeds, 45, 51

O
O blood type, 28
oats, 42, 54, 62, 108, 142
obesity, 52, 90
oestrogen, 63
oils,
    best to use, 62, 100
    frying, 140
    hydrogenated, 62, 65, 66
omega 3
    flax seed oil, 62
    cod liver oil, 62
oranges, 144
osteoporosis, 46, 63
overeating
    carbohydrates, 53, 75
    fats, 65
    proteins, 47

overexercising, 85, 90

P
packed lunches, 125
pancreas, 70, 71, 74
parasites, 137, 151, 157
pasta, 40, 42, 52, 65, 116, 161
peanuts, 40, 129
    O blood type, 28
    B blood type, 32
peppermint tea, 32, 120, 142, 143
phosphorous, 130
pilates, 87
plant based proteins,
    see legumes,
polenta, 60, 95, 99
polyunsaturated fats, 61
potassium, 47, 102, 130, 134
potatoes, 52, 54, 55, 55, 57, 75
potato chips, 40
poultry,
    chemicals in, 137
    A blood type, 30
    B blood type, 32
    O blood type, 28
    AB blood type, 34
processed foods, 62, 65, 114
protein, 72, 73, 75
blood sugar and, 74
brain chemistry and, 74
cheese, 50
daily portions of, 47, 77, 95, 97
deficiency and, 75
eggs, 47, 72, 139
examples of, 97
excess and, 47
fish and shellfish, 50
legumes, 45, 51
meat, 35, 45, 47, 50
nuts, 45, 51
overeating, 47
seeds, 45, 51
soya, 62, 145
vegetarian guidelines and, 45
protein role,
    see muscle mass
    see metabolic rate

Q
quinoa, 42, 60, 95, 141

R
rack of lamb with mustard
    crust recipe, 172
recipes, 166
recommended further reading list, 186
refined foods, avoiding, 53
raw food, 59, 125, 138
reality, living in, 9
restaurants,
    See eating out,
rice, 42, 45, 53, 145
    sugar in, 116
    portions of, 54, 110
roast potatoes, 119
roast turkey thigh with honey
    and ginger glaze recipe, 170
roast vegetables with halloumi recipe, 178
roman cabbage, 175
rooibos tea, 143
rose hips tea, 143
Ross, Julia, 186
rye, 42, 53, 54, 62, 78, 135

S
salmon, 165
salmon en papillote recipe, 173
saturated fats, 73, 77, 135, 140
sandwiches, 125
sausages, 40, 145, 161
sauces, 40, 411, 99, 118, 138
sarsaparilla tea, 143
Sears, Barry, 77
seeds, 45, 51
selenium, 129
Shames, R L and K, 186
Siegel, Bernie, 186
sheeps milk, 42
shellfish, 68
    A blood type, 30
    B blood type, 32
    O blood type, 28
    AB blood type, 34

simple sugars, 52

snacks,
    examples, 102
    necessity of, 101, 118
sleep, 74, 148
    during detox, 37
    extra, 83, 85
soul foods, 115, 117
soya,
    dangers of, 62, 146
    cultural links, 145
spelt, 42, 54, 78, 135, 141, 147
spelt, bread, 185
spelt muffins recipe, 184
spelt pie crust recipe, 184
sports injuries,
    food intolerances and, 147
    kinesiology and, 7
starches, 52, 78, 75, 77
    bad, refined, 60
    good, 56, 60
    portions, 55
    vegetables, 56
stress, 14, 16, 17, 70, 133
sugar, 52
supermarkets, 58, 135, 136
supplements, 129
    See also vitamins, minerals and herbs
support, essential, 10, 17, 18, 93
Swarzbien, Diana, 186
sweeteners, artificial, 100, 126, 134

T

thin, 17
    see underweight
    anorexia, 18
    bulimia, 18
tea, 147
    see food intolerances
        and blood types
    herbal, 142,143
tests,
    candida albicans, 158
    kinesiology, 24
    Nutron, 25
    Thyroid, 156

Vega, 24
The Zone Diet, 77
thyroid, 83, 104, 155
hypothyroid (low), 155
hyperthyroid (high), 163
symptoms of, 156
tests, 155
weight and, 155
thyme tea, 143
transfatty acids, 139
tuna and chickpea salad recipe, 167
tuna curry with coriander and
    coconut recipe, 174
turkey
    see chicken
    roast turkey with honey and
        ginger glaze recipe, 170
turmeric, 130
Type II diabetes, 70, 71
Tyrosine, 131

U

Undereating, 81, 82, 93, 109
Underweight, 18

V

vegetables,
    roast cabbage, 175
roast potatoes, 119
roast vegetables with halloumi, 178
starchy, 57
    unlimited, 56
vinegar
    yeast intolerance and, 40, 100
viruses, 17
    cholesterol and, 68
    obesity and, 147
    selenium and, 129
    wheat and, 147
vitamins,
    B12, 128
    CoQ10, 129
    K, 148

W

walking, 85, 87, 88, 90
water, 38, 102, 118

weight loss graphs, 84
Weil, Dr Andrew, 186
wheat, 148
    alternatives, substitutes, 42
Wild Mushroom and autumn vegetables, 176

Y

yoghurt, 50, 53, 149
yeast overgrowth, 155, 157
yoga, 20, 87
yo-yo dieting, 14, 38, 84

Z

Zone, the, 77
Zzzz's, 149/